Project Management for Health Care Professionals

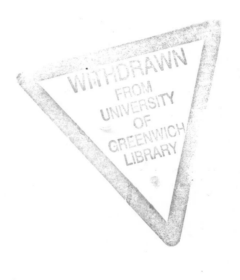

Project Management for Health Care Professionals

Kathleen Roberts and Carol Ludvigsen

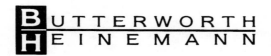

Butterworth-Heinemann
Linacre House, Jordan Hill, Oxford OX2 8DP
225 Wildwood Avenue, Woburn, MA 01801-2041
A division of Reed Educational and Professional Publishing Ltd

A member of the Reed Elsevier plc group

OXFORD BOSTON JOHANNESBURG
MELBOURNE NEW DELHI SINGAPORE

First published 1998

© Reed Educational and Professional Publishing Ltd 1998

British Library Cataloguing in Publication Data
A catalogue record for this book is available from the British Library

Library of Congress Cataloguing in Publication Data
A catalogue record for this book is available from the Library of Congress

ISBN 0 7506 3405 7

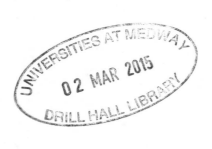

Typeset by E & M Graphics, Midsomer Norton, Bath
Printed and bound in Great Britain by Biddles Ltd, Guildford and King's Lynn

Contents

Introduction

Project Management: some questions and answers

What is Project Management?

A project is a task or undertaking. It is **finite** and usually **time-limited**, involving several stages of work, often with different people. It can come in all shapes and sizes, from building a house, to writing a book, to organizing a conference. It is a process that has a **beginning** and an **end**, a set of **aims** and **objectives** and, ultimately, some specific **outcomes**. Project management is about making a project – any project – happen in an organized way, so as to make best use of **time**, **resources** and **effort**.

Most projects are likely to involve teams of people pooling their skills and knowledge and possibly also their resources; without effective project management, they could be working to different goals with different time scales, lacking the essential resources when these were needed. Project management ensures co-ordination of effort and resourcing, and a focused approach to the task in hand.

How did the idea develop?

The concept of project management began as an area in its own right during the early stages of the American space programme, when a complicated network of scientists, experts and suppliers were engaged in a mammoth exercise involving millions of dollars and vast quantities of equipment. It has since been used in a variety of contexts, especially within industry, where most large construction or manufacturing contracts are 'project managed' down to the last detail.

Now different types of project management approaches have been developed for different sectors of work.

Isn't it extremely complicated and time-consuming?

A plethora of jargon linked to a bewildering range of techniques has developed around project management, such as 'Forcefield Analysis', 'the PICA Cycle', 'SWOT Analysis', 'Gantt Charts' and 'Critical Path Method'. Jargon in this sense is really shorthand; a quick and convenient way of referring to something that people 'in the know' already understand. Some of these techniques may be useful tools for project managers and their organizations, and they will be explained in later sections of this book. They should, however, be regarded simply as tools, to be selected or rejected according to need. No-one contemplating managing a project should allow themselves to be fazed by complicated terminology. One of the purposes of this guide is to de-mystify project management and focus on its essentials.

What about international projects?

Nowadays we live in an international world, where we are part of a European Union of fifteen countries, set to expand even further. Developments which take place on one side of the world at breakfast time are common knowledge on the other by lunch. Within any professional area, colleagues in different countries are able to work together on research and development or on demonstrating or transferring a development, with relative ease.

Nevertheless, everything we do is rooted in our own cultural perceptions, whether in our personal lives or in our work. The way we behave towards our colleagues, the way we dress in the office, the standards we expect at work, are all the results of our experience of living and working in our own particular society. It often doesn't occur to us that things can be radically different elsewhere, and that 'normal' working practices in the UK are far from normal to a Greek, a Dane or a Japanese. The international context in which many projects now operate requires this special consideration if projects are to succeed.

Differences in attitude, perception and working routines are potential minefields when people from different countries are working together on a joint project. Project management in an international context involves building in this knowledge and including strategies for *maximizing* the benefits of cross-cultural co-operation and *minimizing* the risks.

The Structure of the Book

The Guide is in four (unequal) parts. The first section, **Project Management Explained**, sets the scene, outlines the basics of project management, and describes the approaches and techniques used. It also includes a series of appendices on discrete issues like Total Quality Management, Benchmarking and making project applications.

The second part is a **Toolkit** intended to provide project managers and teams with the tools for use in their work. The checklists and 'How to' sheets can be adapted for use in a specific context. Organizations and individuals will need to add or integrate their own criteria or requirements, standing orders or regulations.

The third section, **Project Management for Real**, includes some fairly detailed case studies and examples of real projects based within the healthcare sector.

The final section is the **Jargonbuster** – which speaks for itself.

The overall aim of this book is to give some help to budding project managers. However, there's no substitute for experience, and only one way to really learn. Good luck with your project!

Section 1

Project Management Explained

The mechanics of how to manage projects

The context

The case for using project management techniques

Health services today are particularly concerned with issues such as management of resources, cost containment and standards of customer care. For this reason, systems which assist planning, measurement, resource control and evaluation of success have become widely used. In addition, activities which are externally funded are subject to the requirements imposed by funding agencies, which almost invariably insist on a highly structured approach to planning and delivery.

A project management approach integrates all of these features and is capable of being adapted to fit a diverse range of applications. Initially conceived as a way of controlling and steering very large-scale capital-intensive operations, the techniques involved are equally applicable to small-scale activities and developmental work. Naturally, all projects which are defined as such, will lend themselves to project management. In addition, there will be other kinds of work which are not perceived or identified as 'projects'. Reorganization of a ward or even a waiting area, a survey of patients or service users or a small-scale health education campaign are all examples of activities which would benefit immensely from a simplified project management approach.

Once organizations and individuals have absorbed and integrated the techniques, they become almost second nature.

The public sector and project management

Within the public healthcare sector, a standard project management approach for the introduction of information technology systems was introduced in 1983 as a government initiative. This was redesigned in 1989 to incorporate a number of additional features and was given the name PRINCE.

PRINCE is now in use in most government departments, and many projects which hope to receive government funding will need to adhere to the principles of the PRINCE project management approach. This is a highly-structured system with a complete set of dedicated documentation in the form of five manuals. It has five standard components:

- organization
- plans
- controls
- products
- activities

Tasks are divided into *Technical* and *Management*, and projects are divided into *stages* which have specific outcomes or *products*.

Most of the techniques described in this guide can be easily incorporated into the PRINCE approach, but this book is not a guide to PRINCE (though more information is provided in Appendix 4 which describes it in more detail).

In local authorities, no standard project management system has been imposed, though the principles of Total Quality Management have been steadily gaining ground, and systems like ISO 9000 may be familiar. The rule tends to be that the agency funding (or even part-funding) an activity can impose a structured project management approach if it so wishes – in other words, the piper calls the tune. More usually, it is the format of the documentation which is rigidly imposed on project teams, and there is greater flexibility about the methodologies used for planning, implementation and evaluation.

Project management in an NHS context

The health sector, like every other area of modern society, has been significantly affected by technological changes and advances in recent years. It has also been subject to reorganizations and pressures resulting from higher expectations and increased life expectancy, to name but two factors. One factor alone, the development of what is often called 'the information society', requires healthcare professionals to acquire a whole new set of skills and develop different perceptions and attitudes to their work.

Project management skills may well fall into the category of essential skills for many healthcare staff preparing for the new millennium. Many post-basic professional development programmes offer some insight into project management, but on the whole, the average healthcare professional is lacking in anything more than the basics. Conversely, some staff may have been forced to undertake a project management role without receiving any training in the necessary skills.

The expertise in project management in the health service is often focused in areas like Information Technology, in addition to the aforementioned project managers who have learned how to do it the hard way. It is also probably true that project management ideas have only had any real impact on the health sector in the last ten years, or have been perceived as relevant to the way we provide and deliver health services. However, we are now much more concerned with standards of service, the need for performance indicators and so on, and the concept of value for money. This has resulted in more sophisticated support and monitoring systems being imposed on the health service generally and on project work, and developmental work, in particular. Greater emphasis has also been placed on disseminating the results and outcomes of projects. Publications such as the A–Z reference book were an early attempt at sharing good practice in the NHS.

In 1992, the NHS Executive launched its Information Management and Technology Strategy as a document entitled *Getting Better with Information*. The Strategy described a vision for a better NHS, to be achieved by effective management of information and appropriate use of information technology. The proposal was that all staff should use information to continuously improve their service and the care they provide, thus managing resources more efficiently and saving time and money. The Strategy aimed to encourage sharing of data between organizations in order to achieve:

- more seamless care
- better purchaser/provider relationships

- more efficient and effective contracting
- primary care-led purchasing via the sharing of a common administrative base
- improved administrative systems, e.g. for the ordering of supplies
- access to research and practice-based knowledge to enable the NHS to become more of a 'learning organization'.

The Information Management Group is responsible for leading on the Strategy at national level. The Group produces details of the projects which support the Strategy and which demonstrate how to meet business needs in key areas such as community and direct operational care. It produces a *Programmes and Projects Information Pack* which provides summary reports on all the main programmes and projects currently underway, and is regularly updated. (Available from Information Point/NHS Register of Computer Applications, Information Management Group, NHS Executive Headquarters, c/o Cambridge & Huntingdon Health Authority, Primrose Lane, Huntingdon PE18 6SE.)

Other major policy initiatives

Priorities for improvements to the NHS have been outlined in a series of Government papers which have implications for project management. These include the following:

A Primary Care-led NHS – this White Paper heralded a shift in decision-making within the NHS towards the patients themselves. In a primary care-led service, primary care professionals would be at the centre of a network that would include health authorities and social services, whilst hospital services would assume a supporting role. This document was followed by another, *Choice and Opportunity, Primary Care: The Future*, which proposed that local people should be enabled to develop services that would be more closely matched to their needs and the needs of local services.

The Health of the Nation – set out key areas for action via targets that support health education and health promotion initiatives.

The Patients' Charter – created the need to develop processes of performance monitoring against set standards of service, such as waiting time, etc.

Community Care (Caring for People) – aimed to achieve care in the community at, or close to, people's homes, by securing and delivering integrated care through collaboration with local authorities and other concerned organisations.

Improving cost-effectiveness and maximizing health gain – required an approach which concentrated on the results of healthcare ('does the patient get better?') rather than only looking at the kind of services patients receive. Decisions should be taken on the basis of evidence about clinical effectiveness to determine where resources should be targeted.

The objectives designated in these policy initiatives have provided the impetus for a considerable amount of project work within the healthcare sector. Certainly, all developmental and project-related activity needs to be undertaken within the context set by the initiatives, and government funding is unlikely to be granted to projects which fail to demonstrate such a link. The same principle holds true for other funding agencies, i.e. they will expect any organization in receipt of grant aid to promote their aims and objectives. For example, the European Commission will require projects receiving funding to promulgate EU areas of interest and agreed priorities and may also require them to show that they are providing 'added value' in return for European monies.

Effective project management: more important than ever for the healthcare sector

The drive towards improvements in healthcare services and cost-effectiveness is not only a national preoccupation. Locally too, there is an atmosphere of increased competition amongst NHS trusts and consequently each is eager to demonstrate 'leading edge' practice and to win contracts with local purchasers. Trusts are becoming more diverse and entrepreneurial in their approach to problem-solving and are also aiming to maximize the effectiveness of their human resource strategies. It is often at this level and in these contexts that practitioners first come into contact with project management. Using such an approach can be the ideal way to bring people with different and complementary roles and skills together within organizations. This in turn can help to improve staff cohesion, motivation and morale at a time when organizational change and economic pressures are creating a climate of uncertainty and insecurity.

Project management skills are now in demand in the healthcare sector, as evidenced by the recruitment advertisements in professional journals and magazines. In one edition of the Health Service Journal in January 1997, there were six posts advertised which included project management in their job titles or roles. Courses are now being offered to train staff in project management techniques, including specific training programmes for the PRINCE Government-initiated model of project management.

Different types of projects

There are many different types of projects and many reasons for doing them, for example:

- Solving a problem or addressing a need, e.g. changing duty rotas to meet the needs of women returners.
- Meeting a requirement – possibly imposed by a statutory duty or responsibility, or an internal change of practice, e.g. implementing professional portfolios in line with PREP.
- Testing out an idea or responding to a recommendation – perhaps from an in-house committee, or an idea gleaned from a conference or example of good practice which originated elsewhere, e.g. setting up a European initiative.
- Acting as contractors for an externally-funded and steered project – your organization might have an interest in the area concerned and submit a tender to be involved and do the work, e.g. tendering to provide new community services.
- Following up research and development studies to implement their findings, e.g. implementing new wound care techniques into policy and procedures.
- Trying out improvements to your service, e.g. introducing a new Well Man's Clinic.
- Addressing internal needs – such as organizing a staff development programme within your organization or setting up an information system, e.g. providing staff with training on how to use the Internet.

It may be that these activities have been undertaken before in your organization without the staff concerned consciously using a project management approach. They may have been successful in terms of useful outcomes being produced; however, a more systematic approach ensures that the potential benefits are maximized, and provides the people doing the work with the appropriate tools for the job.

The six stages in brief

Stage 1: developing the project idea

The **idea** is where the project usually begins. It may revolve around a problem to be resolved, or a possible new way of working to be explored, or it may be identified from an external source.

At this initiation stage, it may be fairly vague but the important thing is that it must carry conviction and the originator must be able to communicate it in its essence. Work must be done at this initial point to define the idea clearly and work it up into a presentable form. Whoever does this needs to consider any guidelines/priorities issued by funding bodies or those who will be partners or stakeholders in the project.

Stage 2: assembling the project team

Getting the right mix of people to plan and implement the project is crucial to its eventual success. At this stage, it may only be possible to identify the functions and skills of staff to be involved (or the full team might be recruited if funding is available, or the project has been approved in principle by whoever is funding it)

Stage 3: planning the project

The **plan** is the idea transformed into an organized form. This stage is very important because if any crucial component is omitted, it will probably have a damaging effect during the next stage. Every aspect and phase of the project must be carefully considered and agreed, particularly the aims and intended outcomes. Negotiation needs to take place at this stage on how far partners are prepared to compromise or adapt their original stance. If essential roles are still not filled (i.e., for funding purposes, for addressing gaps in expertise and skills, etc.) progress needs to be made on this as soon as possible. The funding organizations need to be contacted and checks run on deadlines, format of applications, etc. Personal contact (be well briefed prior to meetings!) is always preferable.

Stage 4: making it happen

Implementation is the fourth stage and if project planning has been carried out thoroughly and in sufficient detail, the payoff starts here. Implementation is much more straightforward if all the angles have been covered during the planning stage.

Stage 5: completing the project

Completion is the penultimate stage and the point at which it becomes obvious whether the project has been a success. (At this stage it will become apparent also whether the standards/criteria identified at the start were measurable and useful.)

Stage 6: evaluating the project

Monitoring and **evaluation** of the project need to be considered right from the start and not as an afterthought. Evaluation is crucially important for any project. It must never be omitted, and time and resources must be built in for it whilst the project is being planned. Ongoing evaluation should be built into project implementation, and final evaluation should take place as a discrete stage at the end. Valuable lessons can be learned during this stage, which can feed into future planning and result in much useful intelligence.

(N.B. Some projects may need to include a **dissemination** stage, and this will become clear during the planning of the project.)

As a result of the evaluation stage, there may be a need to apply what has been learned within the organizations involved or even more widely.

N.B. This system of project management has become a familiar model, and owes at least some of its features to the work of Total Quality Management gurus like W. Edwards Deming. See the pages on Total Quality Management at Appendix 2 for more information on this.

The parameters

These will vary given the type of project, but generally will relate to time, cost and qualitative aspects. If a project is externally funded, the funding organization may impose its own parameters. Sometimes these may act as constraints, but whenever possible they should not be perceived or expressed negatively. Parameters provide part of the framework for the project. They must sit comfortably with the goals or objectives and should not act as barriers or obstacles to achieving them, or be seen to be doing so. They will be discussed in more detail in the section on **Stage 3: Planning the project**.

Now to look at the stages in more detail.

Stage 1

The idea

The starting point for every project is the underpinning idea or problem to be addressed.

The validity of this is crucial. There is no point simply having a project for its own sake. And the worst thing anyone can do is to invent a project simply because they think they can get some funding for it (which could then be partially diverted into other activities), though this has been known to happen!

A project comes about because either there is a problem which needs to be solved or because there is an idea to be tested out or developed. It is essential that this basic underlying feature should be made explicit before the project begins.

The origin of the idea or problem

At all stages of project management, clarity is extremely important. The starting point is no exception, and the origin of the project idea needs to be carefully recorded and examined.

There are various ways in which the project idea might have been identified. An individual member of staff or a manager might have proposed it in relation to some research undertaken or feedback gained from service users. It might have been identified as the outcome of a feasibility study or some other preparatory work, which would provide valuable pointers to guide the project planning and delivery. Or it might have been suggested in a strategy group meeting, via quality circles, a patient representative group, or in a team meeting. Whatever the case, there should be a clear statement of how the project idea has been identified and what it is supposed to achieve – its anticipated outcomes.

The idea for the project may have originated outside the UK, for example, staff here may wish to explore whether a model of good practice which has proved successful elsewhere could be transferred or broadened to another context. If this is the case, information about the original project or application should be sought at first hand, in order to avoid any misconceptions about the original work.

Underpinning information and data

The project idea will usually be based on some evidence of need or, at the very least, assumptions made about the problem or issue to be addressed. It is important here to be aware of the potential problems involved in gathering information. For example, when using questionnaires and interviewing people, project team members should be careful not to inadvertently solicit a particular response or to let their own preconceptions and beliefs affect their perceptions. If statistical information or other published material is being used to underpin the project idea, it is a good idea to investigate the context in which the work was undertaken, so as to get an idea of its validity and relevance to the project. It is also important to check when the data was collected to ensure that it is not out of date.

If the project idea is based on a feasibility study or on the recommendations of a previous project, either in-house or external, these should not be accepted at face value but should be re-assessed in the light of any new circumstances.

Initial pitfalls

Lack of clarity is a common pitfall at all stages of project planning and implementation, but it is a particular problem at the stage when the project idea is being defined and developed. If confusion is allowed to creep in now, it will cause difficulties throughout the life of the project and any misunderstandings which develop will cause havoc later. Bias and subjectivity on the part of individual members of staff can also be very damaging.

The best way to ensure clarity of purpose and a common vision is to share information freely and encourage open discussion amongst all those people involved. Record all decisions and make roles and responsibilities clear in notes or minutes, which must be produced quickly after meetings have taken place. Start as you mean to go on.

This commitment to what is often called 'transparency' is particularly crucial when dealing with transnational projects. People in other countries may operate in different ways – in fact, will almost certainly do so and will regard their own style of working as 'normal'. Cultural differences will crop up when least expected and in unforeseen areas; for example, avoid using words like 'urgent' or 'as soon as possible'; always supply a deadline date (and time, if possible) and explain why this is important. If funding is an issue or at risk if people do not meet deadlines, make this plain – it may make your partners leap into action where all other entreaties have failed!

Funding itself is often the greatest problem in project work. This is especially true where a project may require an injection of external funding, which is not available at the initial stages of idea development and project planning. There is simply no way round this, if your organization is unable to commit staffing resources. Many good ideas fail at this stage; convincing others that they should provide development funding for your project is not an easy task. Potential project leaders need to become skilled negotiators at an early stage, and to be able to articulate the unique selling points of their projects clearly and compellingly in order to win over those who hold the purse-strings and the power in their organizations.

Staff involved

At this stage, it is likely that only a small number of staff will be involved and that the project team will not have been assembled. There may also be no formal arrangements for steering or overseeing its progress. However, before undertaking any real work on the project – even the verifying of the idea and gathering of supporting information – care should be taken to ensure continuity of staffing. The people involved now should form the core of the project team, if possible, so that they will feel commitment to the project idea. Simply foisting the work of the project off onto other staff once the planning stage is over and management structures have been set up is unlikely to ensure success.

Identifying the expertise needed for the project is a stage in its own right. Staffing needs will become apparent as the project idea is clarified and defined, and will determine the composition of the project team.

Arriving at agreement

To arrive at a definition of the project, and to identify its aims and objectives, a process of information-gathering and discussion must take place, followed by a broad-brush outline of the project characteristics. This is nothing so definite as planning; that is the next stage, and can begin once the definition of the project is clearer and the project team has been assembled or at least its composition has been identified.

The core team may need to take a day out away from their normal working environment to focus on this task. At the least, they should have a specific meeting to produce the initial project definition and broad aims. **Brainstorming** is a favourite way to do this (see the Toolkit for an explanation of the technique) and can be a useful tool for encouraging people to share and focus on ideas at this and later stages of projects.

By the end of this stage, the following tasks should have been completed:

- gather information and data
- assimilate it and share it as a group
- discuss and clarify issues arising from this
- agree on the definition of the project and its overall purpose
- identify broad, outline timescales for the key stages, staffing needs and other resources required
- identify sources of funding, if not already secured
- list the project imperatives (any absolute 'musts' that need to result from it)
- identify any actions that must be taken to facilitate the planning of the project
- secure management backing and an undertaking to support the project.

Stage 2

The project team

The composition of the project team is crucial to the project's ultimate success. The size of the team obviously depends on the size and complexity of the project, which also defines the amount of time members need to dedicate to the work. A large and complicated project may require full-time staff in addition to people who contribute some of their time and expertise. One which is relatively small-scale and short-term may take up a portion of time from each member of staff involved, working on it in addition to their normal duties. If the latter is the case, ensure that people do not feel they are being pressured into getting involved or feel they are overworked as a result. This is not likely to improve their commitment.

It is also important to ensure that the staff involved have credibility within the organization. The Project Manager or Co-ordinator must have the support of management and access to a line manager at senior level. The Project Steering Group (or whatever mechanism is put in place to provide accountability and overseeing of progress on the project) should be a means of ensuring that all partners are kept informed about the project and have a role in steering it.

Composition of the project team

At the initiation stage of the project when the fundamental idea was discussed, the roles and skills of the team were briefly considered. Some roles and responsibilities are easy to identify and tend to be common to all projects, but others may be specific to your particular activity.

Some common roles are:

- The **Project Manager** or Leader, who is responsible for moving the project forward, co-ordinating the efforts of other staff and exerting overall control, usually working to senior management.
- The **sponsor**, or sponsors, who may be funding the project wholly or in part. Sometimes this might be the organization which has commissioned the project or put the work out to tender (for example, the Department of Health, or a local health authority), or it may be an agency like the European Commission which is providing grant aid for work of a particular nature.
- **Stakeholders** who have some kind of vested interest in the project; they could include **users** of the product or service being developed (e.g. staff or patients) or **suppliers** of materials and technology (e.g., a pharmaceuticals firm). They could also be sponsors.
- **Partners**, who may be contributing funding, expertise or resources to the project. The partnership may be in the form of a **consortium** of organizations and interests.
- The **project team**, consisting of people who have been designated as working on the project.
- **Consultants** or mentors who are providing a designated service or performing an identified function. This could be in the nature of technical assistance or it could be as critical friends, undertaking a role such as monitoring.

Assembling the team

You may be able to assemble your project team from within your own organization or from partner organizations who are also involved. Alternatively, you may need to recruit staff externally to undertake certain roles, and if this is the case, they may not be available until funding is secured and in place.

Whatever the situation, it is imperative that the team has the right mix of **skills**, **experience** and **knowledge** required by the project. In order to decide this, the core team undertaking the initial definition and planning stages of the project need to get together and produce a Project Skills Specification. This can be undertaken as a sub-task in its own right by the core team at this stage, or it can be combined with project planning (the next stage described).

The skills required by the Project Team can be identified in terms of their functions; for example, in addition to any clinical specialisms the team may need, there could be a requirement for an IT specialist, a health promotion officer, or a trainer. There will almost certainly need to be some administrative input and some financial and time management. If the project involves working with transnational partners, there may be a need for language skills or familiarity with the partner culture and way of life.

The Skills Specification is then used as the checklist for ensuring that someone in the project team has the required skills or attributes. If this is not feasible (for example, if some particularly specialised skill is required) then strategies should be identified for securing the skill at an early stage, either from an outside, paid source (such as a consultant) or via links the organization may have which can be exploited for the project's benefit. This means that any budgetary implications can be identified well before the project begins and will not become a stumbling block during implementation.

There is also the issue of project management skills themselves. The skills required for successful project management are varied. Some people have personalities which give them a head start, but others find they have to learn to manage projects from scratch. If this is the case, it can help to undertake some initial staff development activity or training, once you have worked out where your weaknesses lie.

(The self-assessment checklist in the **Toolkit** section helps to define the qualities and skills needed in project management. There is also an example of a Skills Specification sheet.)

Important points which need to be considered when assembling project teams are the **characteristics** and personalities of team members. This is just as important as having the right skill mix. One hyperactive team member with lots of ideas, enthusiasm and drive is fine, but a whole team full of them would be overpowering. The creative, thrusting members need to be balanced by conscientious, thorough people who will provide a steadying influence, and those who are good at getting things up and running need to be balanced by those who meticulously finish a job. Most obviously of all, the team players need a leader who will provide some clear direction and who knows how to manage his or her team so as to get the best out of them.

In addition, the team needs to be **motivated** and **committed** to the project, and members need to feel they are playing a real part in it.

When working out how jobs will be defined and tasks assigned to individuals, try to balance their skills with their characteristics and understand the way in which each person functions best. That is indisputably the way to get the best out of them.

Defining roles and responsibilities

Whether your project team is small or large, all team members must be clear about their roles and responsibilities. These can be agreed initially and reinforced or amended during the life of the project. Regular team meetings, recorded by means of notes circulated to all those involved soon after the meeting, will ensure that there is no confusion about which member of the team is required to take action or to progress any feature of the project. Dates of meetings should be set well ahead to ensure that everyone involved is available.

If external consultants or people from outside organizations are involved, there is a particular need to ensure that work is not being duplicated or omitted. Channels of communication with such people should be set up at the outset of their involvement and regularly monitored.

It may be a good idea to formally identify areas of responsibility and expertise and record them so that everyone involved can have a copy. This will help to define where one person's responsibility ends and another begins, and who is accountable for which resources. A flow chart can also be used in conjunction with this.

If you are the project manager or leader, you will be concerned about the extent of your own accountability and authority. You will usually be required to manage:

- the project implementation procedures and processes
- resources, including staffing
- quality and performance of project deliverables

You may be responsible for monitoring and evaluation, but these tasks are sometimes undertaken by external organizations or colleagues who are not involved with the actual implementation of the project. This is not only to ensure an objective stance, but also brings a fresh viewpoint to the project.

(An example of a Project Management skills checklist is provided at **Toolkit** Sheet 3.)

Steering Committees and other groups

The project team will meet throughout the course of the project, either informally and/or in scheduled meetings. However, it is likely that other colleagues will be involved in the project as members of its steering group or management committee. It is important that they are selected or nominated for their expertise as well as their seniority in the organization, and that they are properly briefed throughout.

The remit of the steering group should also be carefully considered and made explicit. Where it is to approve decisions, the level of these should be made clear, so that the project team's work is not held up on a day-to-day basis waiting for steering group meetings to take place.

Stage 3

Planning the project

During the first stage of work on the project, you discussed the idea or problem to be addressed and defined some of the issues and features of the project in broad terms. Now you will be refining the work undertaken at that stage, thinking in more detail about the work to be undertaken and committing yourselves to a plan of action.

Planning the project in detail can be a lengthy task and no attempt should be made to skimp or save time on this stage. Mistakes made now could be very difficult to rectify later. For example, if a detailed project proposal is being drawn up for a funding agency, errors in calculations or data manipulation could result in serious underfunding or even allegations of fraud. The planning stage is when you will be setting up the systems under which your project will run. Time schedules, budgets, monitoring procedures, quality standards and success criteria are all factors which can help your project to run smoothly – or they can become a headache.

All projects work within fixed parameters and these need to be clearly identified at the planning stage. They may be set by an external funding agency or they may be self-imposed, but they must be realistic and well-defined. **Time, resources** and **quality** are the main factors. Timings in the sense of ultimate deadlines may be imposed on the project by sponsors or funding agencies, but there is usually some flexibility within these to plan the 'internal' deadlines of specific activities and outcomes. Resources are inevitably limited by budgetary considerations, but effective planning can ensure optimum usage and deployment. Quality is a more complex consideration and one requiring careful thought and attention if the project is to be a success and represent value for money.

How to arrive at a plan?

How you actually organize your planning is very much an issue for the individuals involved and the organizational context. Some people may choose to have 'awaydays' so that they can get away from the usual pressures of work and concentrate solely on planning the project, perhaps in a joint event with international partners, if the project is transnational. Others may not be able to do this, or feel it would be of little benefit.

The methods used for arriving at a detailed plan should be chosen or devised with the agreement of the core project team, as far as it has been assembled. There are many methods and techniques that can be used in planning, for example:

- more in-depth brainstorming, with the technique being applied in detail to every stage of the project
- taskboarding – a technique which focuses on establishing the key stages of the project and key tasks relating to them (see the **Toolkit** for a description of this)
- future basing or future planning – a technique developed by a consultancy called ITS (International Training Services), which requires users to develop a 'compelling vision' of what they wish to achieve and work backwards in time from it, establishing exactly how they will realise the vision.

The best advice that can be given in relation to any of these methods is to choose one or more that feels comfortable and appropriate to your needs, and to gain the agreement of the project team rather than imposing a technique upon them. Be careful not to over-complicate matters and if your project is a small and relatively simple one, keep the planning simple too.

All project planning aims to produce some kind of **Work Breakdown Structure**, and involves listing the tasks involved in the project and those required to undertake them. The next stage is to break those tasks down further into their component activities which are split into work packages or separate jobs. All planning techniques work like this, to varying degrees of complexity.

Detailed stages in planning

- Identify all the **partners and stakeholders** involved, secure their involvement and define their roles and responsibilities, then involve them in planning.
- Identify the **aims and objectives** of the project and its **anticipated outcomes and deliverables.**
- Break the project down into individual stages or **milestones** of deliverables; in complex projects, these can also be seen as *work packages*, with a *task* or *work group* being assigned to each one.
- Estimate the overall **timescale**, and the length of time needed for each milestone, taking into account all the critical factors impacting on the project.
- Identify **staffing needs**, including training, for the project as a whole and for each milestone.
- Identify **costs and resource** needs for the project and break these down into needs for each milestone.
- Define **quality standards** for all aspects of the project's work.
- Set **criteria for success** for the project and for milestones.
- Agree a **monitoring procedure** and identify who will be responsible for this.
- Agree a **line management and reporting** structure, including steering groups, etc.
- Plan an overall **evaluation strategy** for the project, including formative and summative evaluation.
- Plan a **dissemination** and feedback strategy (if applicable).
- Summarize the above into an **implementation plan** or work breakdown structure which should be copied to all those involved.
- Produce an overall budget for the project.

Aims, objectives and anticipated outcomes

These have been broadly agreed at Stage 1. Now you will have to make a commitment to them, so you may wish to look at them in the light of the other features of your project. For instance, are they achievable given the time and resources available or should they be amended slightly?

Partners and stakeholders

These may be colleagues from similar organizations in other countries or from complementary organizations, who can bring an extra dimension to the project, or add value in some way. The purpose and extent of their involvement needs to be made explicit now, and agreement secured from them that they will undertake the tasks required. If external funding is being sought (for example, from a European Union programme) this involvement may need to be formally documented before a project proposal can be submitted.

It is a good idea to agree the frequency of meetings and arrangements for hosting and recording these with partners at this stage, as there may be staffing and cost implications for them. It goes without saying that you need each partner organization to nominate an individual member of staff with whom you can work, and to whom all communications can be addressed. Organize a meeting involving all these people as soon as possible, and try to include some kind of social activity or ice-breaking session, so that easy working relationships can be established.

Milestones or work packages

Each step or individual stage of your project needs to be mapped out and delineated in terms of its tasks and its particular outcomes. These 'milestones' are discrete blocks of work which can be plotted and allocated time schedules of their own. This is a useful way of breaking large projects down into manageable chunks and also of measuring progress more easily. Each milestone can have its own recorded tasks, objectives and success criteria and these can be itemized on a milestone sheet (an example is provided in the Toolkit).

Milestones can be assigned their own individual budgets, and where work is being contracted out (for example, to consultants) payments can be geared to milestone completion.

In a large and complex project, you may need to break down the totality beyond milestones and into detailed work packages, each with a list of objectives and tasks, and final deliverables. A Work Breakdown Structure should be completed for each work package showing what needed to be done and the resources required, etc. A work group or task group will then be made responsible for that particular work package, with members meeting independently of Project Team meetings. Each member of staff might be part of several work groups, depending on their skills and time commitment to the project.

However, remember that your project management systems are there to *facilitate* your work – don't make the mistake of setting up very complicated systems for a small and relatively-easily managed project; the rule is to keep it simple!

Timescales

These need to be realistic enough for everyone involved to feel they can meet deadlines within the time available, and flexible enough to accommodate slippage and unforeseen delays. There are mathematical formulae for calculating timescales but they are of limited use, and the best way is to use your commonsense and negotiate deadlines with team members involved, based on their own experience.

A useful strategy for checking timescales is to go through the planning process, working forwards, until you have completed the process. Then check the feasibility of the deadlines you have imposed, or which have been imposed upon you, by working *backwards* from them. Use a calendar and plot all the critical factors which have a timescale implication, including organizational commitments, public holidays, staff training events, etc. and always allow more time than you feel you need to complete a task. Check out your timescales with others. In most organizations, there are people who are known to be particularly skilled at time management; ask them for advice on your timetables and involve them as internal consultants if they are willing.

Don't forget to allow time at the end of the project for completing returns or reports for sponsors and funding agencies – this can be time-consuming and complicated, but is an essential part of the project workload.

Staffing needs

You may already have carried out the Skills Specification exercise mentioned earlier, as part of the project team development stage. (If not, you may want to do it now as part of the planning process.) This should be helpful in identifying the staff mix you require, and also in pinpointing staff development and training needs. Now you can specify these for each milestone, so that staff are recruited well in advance, have been trained and have time to practise their newly-acquired skills before they will be tested.

Identifying staffing needs for each milestone helps to focus the human resource management aspects of your project. In very complex projects, there may be a need to bring in different specialists at different points of the project lifespan, and these can be mapped out so that the resource and time implications are clear before implementation begins. Staffing costs are often the most expensive budgetary heading, so it is important to estimate them as accurately as possible.

Resources and costs

This includes everything from the actual money required to pay for additional costs relating to the project, to the equipment, office space and staff needed to ensure it is adequately resourced. If you are lucky and the project is being supported from within your organization, from a single department, you may simply be allocated resources on a goodwill basis without having to account for them in detail. But the more likely scenario is that there will be a proportion of external funding involved, and that the agency providing it will require detailed accounts and budgets identifying all the resources dedicated to the project. Many organizations now operate a system of cost centres, and one section or department may in effect provide services to another at an identified charge.

The expertise and knowledge of your finance officer will be invaluable when costing out your project, and he or she should be involved at an early stage. You will need to agree or arrive at a series of headings under which costs will be itemized – this will usually be imposed upon you by your own organization's budgetary procedures or by the body providing external funding.

You may be applying for funding for your project from one of the European programmes available to support developmental work and training activities. In such cases, it is usual that any externally-provided grant aid must be 'match-funded' by your organization and its partners, to a specified percentage formula. If this is so, you should read the guidance issued in relation to the programme concerned with care, as it will specify any existing resources which can be included in the costings as your contribution to the project budget. If in doubt, contact the programme support unit, who will be able to advise on allowable costs. Never assume that some costs (such as equipment and building hire) are going to be covered by external funding – always check first that they are eligible under the programme concerned.

Take care when estimating costs to include a percentage increase for future years, if your project will span more than the current one. It may also be necessary to include amounts for depreciation of equipment; your finance officer should be able to advise on this. If your project is transnational or EU-funded, be prepared for currency fluctuations and make sure you keep up to date with the value of the Euro (as this is how the European Commission will pay your grant aid).

If you are not required to complete an application form including specified project costings (for example, if your project is an in-house operation) you should still itemize your resource needs and costs.

One way of bringing all your resource needs together for planning purposes is to use a resource identification summary sheet, like the one provided in the **Toolkit**. It can always be modified at a later date, but is a useful way of identifying all resource needs in one go.

Quality standards

Quality is an issue which comes to the fore at this stage of planning, but it should be obvious by now that any worthwhile system of project management is steeped in a quality culture. The underlying premise of TQM (Total Quality Management) is about getting a process and its products as fault-free as possible, and of making continuous improvements thereafter. (For more information, see Appendix, p. 64.)

A great deal of project work is developmental and innovative rather than repeatable – it may involve creating a model or exemplar, testing a theory, undertaking research, or transferring good practice to a new context. Your project is essentially the final performance, rather than a rehearsal, so you need to get it right first time. Aim for the absolute best you can achieve within the resources available and expect no less. Conversely, don't allow yourself to be saddled with quality standards that are simply unrealistic given the context in which you are operating. Apply quality standards to *all* aspects of your work, including any documentation circulated or publications produced, and define these at the planning stage so that they are fixed at the outset.

It is essential when doing this to be clear about what you mean by quality. Some definitions rely on phrases like 'fit for the purpose intended' or 'at a level which will satisfy the customer's requirements'. These are really only intended as a starting point and will need to be made more specific in order to be translated into applicable criteria – in other words, to provide standards that are measurable. For example, in the case of project documentation, the quality standards agreed might include:

Clarity – documents are easy to read, all the words are legible and written in a clear style which conveys meaning fluently and accurately.

Presentation – documents are complete, laid out according to house style, with pages in order and numbered.

Many organizations have TQM teams made up of staff responsible for research and development, audit, practice development, etc. These can be consulted and involved in the project, if they are willing.

However, if your organization does not already have a quality system in place, you may need to introduce one which has been devised for the project, and train staff accordingly. For example, clerical or administrative staff working with the project team can be trained and then asked to be responsible for a range of items, such as the quality of all documentation issued, and the maintenance of project records. Initially, you may have to institute a system of checklists to monitor the standards, but after a time it will become second nature to staff to work to the levels defined. Take care at this point not to rest on your laurels – this is not a time to discard the old checklists but to agree new ones with the team which take your standards of work even higher.

Criteria for success

When you know what you are aiming to achieve in terms of outcomes or deliverables, both at the level of individual milestones and for your project as a whole, you need to have a clear idea of their success criteria. These provide you with the tools for assessing and measuring what has been achieved. The success criteria you identify will vary from project to project. Some projects are concerned with producing concrete outcomes such as physical objects (e.g. a new department or building) which must be capable of functioning under certain conditions, and the success criteria for these, or for this part of the work, are usually straightforward. Others may be more complex or 'woolly', and require thoughtful definition. Even relatively straight-forward data-related projects, such as establishing a new patient record and appointments system, can be far more complex than they initially appear, once both users and providers have articulated their needs and requirements. The success criteria should be tailored to the individual project and not simply tacked on as general statements.

The criteria themselves tend to be either quantifiable ('hard') or qualitative ('soft').

Quantifiable criteria tend to be things which can be specified in physical terms or in relation to recognized standards, such as:

- involving specified numbers of people in the project
- meeting deadlines or achieving outcomes within defined timescales
- staying within agreed cost or other resource limitations.

Qualitative criteria are much less tangible and less oriented towards 'number crunching'. They often require more sophisticated or subtle forms of measurement, and might include such factors as:

- aesthetic improvements
- changes in attitude and perception
- awareness-raising and consciousness-raising.

Be careful how these are phrased – avoid woolly or subjective words – and ensure that they are always measurable in some way (you may have to devise one specifically).

Some success criteria will be easy to identify, whilst others will need more deliberation. It is important to involve everyone in the process as far as possible. Some stakeholders may have their own ideas about success criteria and these may have to be accommodated, but never allow assumptions to be made about this crucial area; again, be absolutely clear and unequivocal and record all decisions accurately.

Monitoring procedures

Once you have identified your success criteria, you need to devise ways of getting at the information you need for applying it. Some data may be easy to access (e.g. numbers of people seen at an out-patient clinic in any one day) whilst some may be more tricky (views and perceptions of patients using the clinic). The methodology used to gather this information may affect how reliable or useful it is, so bear this in mind when planning. It may be useful to involve staff with expertise in data collection and make use of their expertise, for example, in phrasing questionnaires and organizing surveys.

Monitoring is basically the process of using your already-defined criteria for success to measure progress and achievements. Monitoring procedures can be external, internal or preferably a mixture of both. Each milestone should be subject to on-going monitoring to ensure that progress is on course. Do not wait until the end of the milestone period to find out that you have overspent on your budget allocation, for example. Identifying slippage or the need for readjustment at an early stage usually means that a situation can be salvaged, so a good monitoring system must be in place before the project gets off the ground. Plan exactly how progress will be monitored and by whom, for each stage or milestone, and make this explicit in your documentation.

The project will also need to be monitored as a whole, but breaking it down into separate milestones and monitoring these individually helps to maintain tight control whilst work is in progress. Monitoring also provides the information required for the process of evaluation.

Monitoring techniques used on their own are not much use unless the information gained is communicated to the course team and other concerned individuals in feedback. Methods devised for monitoring should ensure that it is possible to feed information back rapidly, rather than in the form of long, beautifully produced reports that are submitted too late to act upon. In addition to the monitoring methods selected for your individual project, you will probably be required to use the usual methods for reporting on progress and ensuring accountability which are accepted as the norm in your organization, or imposed by your funding agency. These are likely to include team meetings, Steering Group meetings with regular progress reports, presentation of data on success criteria, etc.

Don't forget to allow time for monitoring within your own work-load, so that you are able to make monitoring visits to other sites, have meetings with staff based outside the office, etc.

Line management and reporting structures

All organizations have a line management structure and both internal and external accountability and reporting procedures, though their effectiveness is variable. Projects are a microcosm of organizations in this sense, and large-scale, public funded ones will have to build in a proportion of time and resources to this.

When planning your project, bear in mind how best this can be done. Try to ensure that the people nominated or selected to your steering group are knowledgeable and committed, and will make a real contribution rather than simply rubber-stamping or vetoing proposals put to them. Draw up a notional schedule of meetings so that progress can easily be made; for example, if your organization's management team is required to approve certain actions or budgetary expenditure, ensure that you are aware of their timetable of meetings.

Consider the remit of the different groups and individuals involved in the accountability and reporting structure and draw up terms of reference for groups to be agreed at the first meeting. If the reporting structure is complex, draw up a diagram showing how groups and individuals inter-relate. Ensure that this is displayed in the project team's office or circulated to team members, and also included in any briefing packs prepared for steering group members.

Evaluation

Many people think that evaluation is an activity carried out at the end of a project and that no serious thought need be given to it until then. This is a mistake. The evaluation plan needs to be worked out before the project begins, and should include formative as well as summative evaluation procedures.

Formative evaluation is undertaken during a project or activity and is tied into the monitoring process. The information gained from monitoring enables judgements to be made about how the project is going in terms of how well you are progressing towards your goals. For instance, monitoring of milestone achievements means that you can continually reassess your progress against the original aims and objectives identified to ensure that these are realistic and achievable, and modify or amend them as necessary whilst the project is still underway. An effective formative evaluation system enables fine adjustments to be made, rather like retuning an engine in order to get the best performance out of it.

Summative evaluation is an assessment carried out at the end of the project and will be discussed in more detail later in a section in its own right. However, various actions will have to be taken in advance of the final evaluation procedure in order for it to work effectively, and these need to be identified at the planning stage. (For example, the selection of a sample of respondents to give you feedback, the devising and printing of questionnaires, etc.) If your success criteria were carefully chosen and appropriate, and applied properly by your monitoring procedures, you should have the right kind of information (and in sufficient quantity) by the end of the project for judgements to be made about its impact and effectiveness.

Feedback from project team members, service users and project beneficiaries is often the most valuable ingredient of the evaluation process. The use of an external evaluator such as a consultant, who can provide an objective perception, is also strongly recommended. Getting roles and responsibilities clear from the outset is imperative, and written specifications should be produced and circulated to ensure that team members understand the system and its associated procedures.

In addition, time should be built into the project timetable to allow for any beta testing or assessment of prototypes, and for making the modifications that may be necessary following such an exercise.

Whilst you are planning the evaluation of your project, you need to re-examine exactly what it is that you are planning to produce at the end of the project. What are your intended outcomes? Are there any secondary outcomes which are desirable but not absolutely essential? What are the characteristics of the product of the project? For example, you may be aiming to produce something innovatory in terms of practice. How are you going to evaluate the innovatory aspects of your outcomes – and how will you know that they are really innovatory?

Draw up a simple diagram or list of project outcomes and their characteristics. Some of the latter may be dictated by your sponsor or funding agency, for example:

innovatory
transferable
value for money
commercially viable
involving real transnational partnerships, not just on paper.

Decide how you are going to evaluate these and what needs to be done in order to do this.
(See **Stage 6: Disseminating and evaluating the project**)

Dissemination

If your project is likely to produce something which would be beneficial to other organizations or individuals, you should plan to disseminate information about it widely. There is always the danger that the same or similar developmental work is being done in a variety of settings and being unnecessarily duplicated, thus wasting resources. Also, important breakthroughs or improvements on practice may pass unnoticed if they are not disseminated.

Dissemination can take a variety of forms, but like every other project component, it has resource implications so it should be thought out at the planning stage of the project. You may choose to disseminate information about your project during its lifespan, or wait until it has been completed. On-going dissemination is often the better option, if budgets and timescales allow, and where you have a number of transnational partners the dissemination programme will have to span several countries. Whenever you do it, you need to ask the questions 'why?', 'what?', 'how?', 'when?' and 'who?', before you start.

Dissemination methods can include:

- newsletters and bulletins
- events like conferences, seminars and workshops, or inputs to them
- articles in journals and professional publications
- use of the Internet and World Wide Web (via news groups or your organization's Web page).

Some of these may cost nothing but staff time, others may involve a charge to your project budget, whilst others (like a dissemination conference) may perhaps be income-generational. All will need to be built into the project budget and implementation plan. Sometimes project evaluation and dissemination can be usefully combined. For example, a network of people can be involved in providing feedback on project outcomes during the lifespan of the project, and can assist with dissemination by cascading it to their own networks.

At the planning stage of your project, you should work out your dissemination strategy at least in outline. Make it flexible enough to cope with changes of plan or adjustments to project outcomes, and 'revisit' it during the project lifespan to make these amendments rather than wait until the final dissemination phase, that is, dissemination of project outcomes, comes into play.

Be prepared to keep records of all dissemination activities. If your project is EU-funded, the European Commission may require an account of your dissemination programme with a log of the activities involved.

The Implementation Plan

All of these component parts can be summarized into an implementation plan which depicts the overall structure of the project. There are various ways of doing this, some based on a written narrative, others on flow charts or other graphical illustrations (one example is provided in the **Toolkit**). Select a method you and your team feel appropriate to your project and to the way you work. The main concern is to ensure that the method chosen allows for the *totality* of the project to be grasped – by now you may all feel that you 'can't see the wood for the trees' anymore.

This is the time when you might notice that something has been left out of your planning, and you should be able to identify which milestone stage it will fit into, and rectify the omission. The project budget can now be summarized too, and scrutinized in its entirety. (There is a separate note in the Appendices on costings.)

Stage 4

Making it happen

You have now arrived at the point where your meticulous planning is about to pay off. Everyone in the project team is starting the implementation phase with a shared vision of the project and a full set of documentation mapping out how you are going to proceed. In addition, you will have established a system of working together and keeping each other informed so that progress can be made and monitored, and any necessary amendments to the original plan can be made quickly and easily.

Everyone will have copies of the project proposal, the implementation plan, the schedules agreed for each milestone, their agreed roles and responsibilities and any flow charts or diagrams produced to steer the project's progress. They will also have copies of the budgets agreed, the regulations in place governing use of resources and expenditure and the schedule of project team meetings and other timescales.

Now is the time to ensure that there is an effective **control system** in place, which will operate throughout the implementation stage and help you to keep the project on course. It is important to be clear about the role of such a system; it is not put in place to control the project itself, but to act as a facilitating mechanism enabling the project manager and team to monitor and control progress.

The aim is to establish and maintain a process which enables you to:

- gain an accurate picture of what is actually happening
- measure this against what was originally planned to happen
- identify the areas of divergence and assess whether these need to be

corrected (in some instances, what is happening may be an improvement over what was planned!)
- decide what action needs to be taken
- implement the decision.

The control system should be concerned specifically with:

- **Time management** – so that tasks are being undertaken as planned and objectives achieved, and that project outcomes are being delivered as agreed.
- **Resource and cost management** – ensuring that resources required are in place when needed, and that over- and underspending is avoided.
- **Quality management** – making regular checks on the quality of on-going work and on the quality of outcomes.
- **People management and interaction** – ensuring that staff have the right mechanisms for effective communication, are performing well and working to their potential, and have established and maintained good working relationships.
- **Feedback and corrective action** – providing feedback on the above four components, so that any problems can be quickly identified and changes made accordingly. Similarly, such feedback enables good practice in one area of the project to be identified and transferred.

The systems used should be as simple as possible. The people using them should feel that they own and are in control of them, rather than the other way round. Procedures used should not be so rigid that they cannot be changed or amended; projects are dynamic things which are by their natures developmental. To learn the most from them and derive the greatest benefit, we need to be prepared to develop with them. Your project control system should be flexible enough to take account of this and also to cope with contingencies such as staff illness, organizational change or external pressures.

Critical factors

Before systems can be put in place for controlling the project during implementation, it is necessary to define exactly *what* is being monitored and controlled. The broad areas are as stated above, but each project is individual and has its own critical factors. There will also be a range of known factors which will have some effect on the project and will have to be taken into account, such as holiday periods, financial year endings and other occurrences. Most of these will have been identified during the planning stage, but regular, 'looking ahead' checks need to be made during implementation to ensure they are all foreseen, and any new ones identified as soon as possible.

Critical factors can be internal to the project – and therefore within your control to a large extent – or external, so that you may not be able to control them. The latter may include factors such as:

- A planned development or innovation being in place at the right time, for example, a new computer system, getting onto the Internet or using email.
- Additional or differently-skilled human resources within the organization, such as the recruitment of new members of staff.
- An increase or cut in budget.
- Partners withdrawing from the project (especially difficult if it is a transnational activity).
- The information required by sponsors or funding bodies by the end of the project, which may not be known at the outset.

Plenty of notice is needed on all critical factors and though some may be outside your control, try to take steps to minimize their potential for disruption. In the case of the last example, it is essential to have some idea of what will be required as soon as possible. In some instances, the funding agency may ask for data which you have simply not collected or ask for it to be presented in a way that is completely new. If the agency has not provided blank forms for end-of-project returns by a stage halfway through the project, or they are not expected until nearer the conclusion, contact them and ask informally what they are likely to require.

All critical factors need to be taken into account and contingencies devised in case they do not materialize as envisaged. Similarly, there will be critical factors in your own project work, planned by yourself, for example:

- ordering and installation of new equipment or software which has been designated for the project
- staff training and development in relation to the project

- the timescales and deadlines you have set for completion of milestones and production of deliverables or outcomes.

In the planning stage, it was possible to identify all of these in the key stages in which they occurred, plot them and prepare for them, and then work *backwards* from them to ensure that the project team would have the time and resources available to cope with them. During implementation you will discover how accurate your estimates were, and how successful were your efforts to build in flexibility to your project management.

Project management is people management

As a project manager or leader, your role may be essentially supervisory. Individual team members may be undertaking the specific workaday tasks of the project, whilst you oversee their work and co-ordinate their efforts. You need to make sure that they are working together smoothly, and using all the methods put in place to ensure effective cross-communication. At the same time, you don't want team members to feel you doubt their competence and are checking their work for suspected mistakes all the time.

It is easy for friction to arise between team members, especially in large-scale projects where staff are divided into task groups, who may feel they are in competition or being compared with one another, perhaps critically. If you have not managed groups of people before, it is worth giving this some thought before embarking on the 'real' work of the project, and either undertaking some specific training in negotiation and people management or at least doing some reading on it. Some useful pointers are:

- **Develop self-awareness** – make sure you understand your own strengths and weaknesses and have a reasonably accurate self-image. At the same time, be aware of how other people perceive you and ensure that your behaviour does not give them confusing or erroneous messages
- **Be aware of the nature of stress** – a challenge is one thing, but an overdose of stress can cause serious emotional and physiological reactions. Don't allow yourself or your team members to get to this point. Effective and supportive communication (talking to people!)

and time management are two simple precautions which can be taken from the start of any project or activity.

- **Look at problems creatively** – there are often ways of solving apparently insoluble problems, if you can look at them imaginatively and with a really open mind. Some problems can act as catalysts or actually produce benefits for individuals or organizations if treated in this way.
- **Develop motivating skills** – this is obviously a lot easier if you are motivated yourself!
- **Manage conflict without blame** – the key to this is to isolate problems, not people. In any position where there is a conflict of opinion or a breakdown in negotiation, don't personalize it – identify the problem and get all parties to tackle that, not each other.

Above all, be prepared to listen to other team members and colleagues and respect their opinions.

Making the most of meetings

Meetings can often be perceived as a waste of time, particularly when they have become such fixtures in the routine of an organization or unit that they take place as a matter of course. They have become so much a part of life that we rarely consider their functions or ensure that they are fulfilling these.

It is worth reminding ourselves that meetings take place so that things can happen which could not otherwise be achieved, involving specific groups of people. It is also worth calculating the cost of a routine meeting in terms of the staff time and travel involved – depending upon the seniority and numbers of people concerned, it will probably amount to anything from £500 to £1000, possibly more. Add to that the fact that the people involved in the meeting would have been doing other productive work (at least in theory!) if they had not been attending, and the conclusion must be that meetings should be made to earn their place in the project timetable.

In fact, well-planned, properly conducted meetings are essential both to project planning and to implementation, and fulfil a range of important functions. These include:

- decision-making
- recording of decisions and responsibilities

- reporting on progress
- monitoring of progress and other factors
- problem-solving
- reviewing and evaluating
- forecasting and planning.

All managers have the authority to take certain day-to-day decisions individually, without recourse to a steering group, and any who feel unable to take decisions will soon lose credibility with their teams. But many decisions are best taken within groups, not just so that responsibility is shared, but because different people bring different perspectives to bear upon an issue, and are more effective in solving problems or being creative than one person acting alone.

Work can be progressed via meetings when tasks are interrelated or interdependent, and staff can use the meeting forum to agree the basis for handing over responsibility or providing mutual support. They also have a monitoring function in that task group leaders or staff responsible for certain activities can report on progress and alert the rest of the team to any slippage or other problems. In addition, meetings act as a networking mechanism to identify good practice and transfer it to other areas of the project.

It is important that meetings are adequately recorded. Minutes or notes should be well-written but brief and to the point, with a clear statement of actions agreed and who is to progress them. It goes without saying that the notes should be circulated to everyone who needs them as soon as possible after the meeting.

When working with groups and committees, you need to bear in mind their **Terms of Reference**. During the planning process, you considered the remit of any steering committees or other groups relating to the project carefully, and drew up terms of reference for them which outlined their role and responsibilities. Now you need to ensure that these groups adhere to their remits and that there is enough flexibility to widen or amend them if the need arises.

Some guidelines for managing meetings

(This is not a book about managing meetings; there is already a plethora of such publications from which readers can take advice, and many experienced staff might well feel affronted at the suggestion that they need such advice anyway. But meetings are an important part of the management process and a brief note on their organization and control can be used as an aide mémoire if nothing more.)

When **organising or calling meetings**, take care to:

- Give as much notice of the date(s) as possible – so that people have room in their diaries and have time to prepare properly.
- Make clear the purpose of the meeting and the actions or decisions which need to be taken.
- Check domestic or other practical arrangements – availability of rooms, equipment you need to use including audiovisual aids, support facilities, etc.

Prior to the meeting

- Send out a short agenda with supporting documentation. Make sure this documentation, and the subsequent record of the meeting, is produced to quality standards (see the checklist in the **Toolkit**) and contains all the information necessary.
- Meet with, and fully brief the person chairing it, if this is not yourself.
- Make arrangements for it to be recorded, if this has not already been done.

During the meeting, ensure that:

- It starts punctually and stays on course, finishing within the time allowed.
- All decisions which need to be taken have been processed and that all those involved have understood them.
- The discussions which take place are relevant and fruitful (a good Chairperson will curtail any that are going nowhere).
- Previous decisions taken or tasks assigned are checked on and progressed further.

After the meeting, check that:

- A record of it has been written up into notes which accurately summarize the decisions taken and any other important points made or issues raised. This should also include the date of the next meeting.
- The correct procedure for approval of minutes is being followed, if applicable (this is usually that they are sent to the Chairperson for agreement).

- The minutes or notes have been sent out promptly and circulated to the right people.
- Meeting records are being maintained in the files.
- People in the team are reading the notes and acting upon them where appropriate.

Using the control tools prepared

The project has been plotted at the level of depth and complexity required, and an appropriate control system has been devised to ensure that it stays on course. You now need to sharpen up the tools you selected and put them into practice.

Within your control system, it is important to get into the habit of on-going monitoring from the outset of the implementation stage, so that it becomes a way of life, and team members feel comfortable with it. This can be done relatively easily by building it in to the project routine, for example:

- Initiate a routine of short, informal team meetings at the end of each week where members give rapid oral progress reports. Encourage people to share concerns about possible threats to deadlines or deliverables immediately they are suspected, so that contingencies can be devised. The inaugural meeting should take place just before implementation begins and should include a recap of the project's organization and procedures.
- Make regular monitoring visits to any remote sites to check on progress and ensure that staff based there do not feel isolated.
- Use all means available (telephone, fax, email) to maintain regular communication with any colleagues at a distance (e.g. transnational partners) and meet as frequently as budgets and time constraints allow.
- Be open about all monitoring methods and display documentation such as checklists and charts on a team noticeboard.
- Encourage team members to monitor their own work and tasks in progress and to evaluate it critically (they can only do this in an atmosphere of supportive and positive criticism).
- Create an environment in which errors or breakdowns can be identified objectively and without blame, so that it becomes possible to discuss how failures might have been avoided, and integrate

improvements to systems. Be open about your own errors of judgement in a matter-of-fact way, as an example to team members.

Controlling costs

Your overall project budget was identified at the planning stage, as were the mechanisms for funding it, and for recording expenditure. If your organization has a Management Information System this would probably take care of the latter, but you may have been required to set up a separate control system or account by the funding agency supplying grant aid to your project.

You also arrived at detailed cost breakdowns for the separate work packages or milestones of your project, and one reason for doing that was to facilitate the task of monitoring expenditure. The monitoring of expenditure and of all financial aspects of the project must be very tightly organized during implementation so that any divergence in this area will be spotted straight away. Underspending can be almost as much of a problem as overspending in certain circumstances, so make sure that the questions asked or procedures used are able to identify this.

Any monitoring of project costs and resources should include the following components:

- Communication with and supervision of staff responsible for financial control and accounting.
- Inclusion of cost and resource monitoring in regular team meeting agendas.
- Scrutiny of actual account documentation or spreadsheets (which may need explanation by accounts staff).
- On-going monitoring procedures such as the use of simple checklists (like the one in the **Toolkit**).
- Spot checks or a 'dummy audit' to ensure that staff are adhering to the procedures laid down for project expenditure and record-keeping.

One common problem which may arise with externally-funded projects is that they are subject to a different set of regulations and procedures for financial management and accounting. The organization's own staff will naturally be familiar with internal procedures and will be unaware of any others unless they are properly briefed.

This should have occurred at the planning stage but must be continually reinforced during implementation, starting with the first project team meeting. Regular checks must be made to ensure that staff understand the procedures fully. In the event of staff time being an accountable resource (for example, where staff may have been seconded part-time to the project or are simply spending part of their time on it), a timelogging system will need to be established and monitored. As staff time may have been costed into the budget and may well be the most expensive item, it is important that it is accurately monitored.

Monitoring quality

The quality standards which were considered acceptable for working practices and project outcomes were identified during the planning stage. During implementation, these must be particularly carefully monitored; quality is probably the most critical aspect of all, because if the work your team produces is below standard, and the outcomes produced are not fit for their purpose, the whole project has been a waste of time and resources. If any lapses in quality occur, or work falls below the standards identified, early notification gives you the best chance of taking corrective action.

However, the monitoring of quality is an area which can be problematic. When you and your team defined your quality standards, you would have been at pains to make them clear and specific. Now you may find that it is often possible to disagree about the meaning of a word or interpret it in different ways, especially where there are vested interests. When quality standards were considered earlier, documentation was used as an area where quality standards would apply, and words like 'clear' and 'easy to read' were used in the example. Personal styles of writing differ so widely that it is not hard to imagine considerable dissension arising on these points alone. During the early stages of implementation it is as well to allow time for discussion in order to arrive at conscious agreement on the range of quality criteria established.

Similarly, there may be disagreement during monitoring on the **criteria for success** defined for measuring the project's progress and achievements. Again, the best strategy is to work through the areas of difficulty at an early stage and negotiate agreement. If you are using external monitoring, the consultant or 'critical friend' undertaking this role will be able to act as an arbiter to some extent. Ultimately, if team members do not agree on issues, you as project leader may need to step in and make a final ruling.

Dealing with divergence

The monitoring systems you have in place should ensure that you are rapidly alerted to any divergence from your original plan, such as slippage in the project timescale. Any variation from planned activity should be carefully noted by the staff concerned and reported to the team or to the project manager if there is no immediate team meeting planned. The divergence should be carefully examined and unless it is agreed to be insignificant, subjected to a review procedure. This should involve asking a series of key questions such as:

- how does this affect:
    the project timescale and deadlines?
    the budget?
    the objectives?
    the deliverables?
    staffing and resources?
- do any of the above need to be modified?
- how can this be done with the least disruption?
- can contingency plans/funds cope?
- is the divergence such that some parts of the project may have to be cancelled or aborted?
- is the whole project at risk?
- should management be informed of the problems?

and so on. This can be done as a team exercise. At the same time, add some questions that are positive, for example:

- are there any beneficial effects resulting from this, including 'hidden' benefits?
- what can we learn from it?
- can we view it creatively and with an open mind?

In the event of a divergence going undetected until it has become a real problem, you may need to hold a specific team session to unravel the complexities and work out what went wrong.

Don't look back in anger, use a Total Quality Management technique!

When your project hits a snag, as it almost certainly will, you need to analyse what went wrong so that similar mistakes can be avoided in the future. The essential factor here is to remove the feelings of blame and guilt which can be so damaging to effective working relationships. People who feel they are being blamed for a mistake and will be punished for their error are unlikely to admit it openly whilst there is still time to take remedial action. They may even try to hide the mistake or put the blame onto other colleagues.

The trick here is to make a clear separation between responsibility and blame. Encourage staff to take *responsibility* in the knowledge that they will be helped and supported, and given credit for the level of autonomy and professionalism that this indicates; treat the idea of *blame* with disdain as a non-productive and negative concept. Ensure that you demonstrate this, rather than simply preach it, or you will lose credibility with your team.

Tools and techniques for analysing what went wrong are also useful because they help to de-personalize the issue. It is possible to turn a disaster into a team-building exercise by having a session on plotting how a mistake occurred, and identifying all the contributory factors, at the same time highlighting how these could have been avoided or remedied. (Don't overdo this, however; team members will soon get tired of having a post-mortem after every mistake.) Be aware of people's sensitivities when conducting such meetings, and if possible, bring in a consultant or trained externally-based member of staff to run one as a workshop initially. This means that the technique is introduced by someone who is not in a position of authority over team members, who may be feeling raw about their errors.

One such technique for unravelling fairly complex mistakes or problems is by using a Cause and Effect Diagram, sometimes also called a Fishbone Diagram because its shape resembles a fish's skeleton. (An example is provided in the **Toolkit**.) It can be used for other purposes, such as a second-stage planning tool for taking brainstorming ideas a step further on or evaluating ideas produced during such a session.

Taking corrective action

Once you have worked out what went wrong, why and what the implications are, you may need to take corrective action. Depending upon the nature of the problem or the degree of divergence, this may not be an onerous task. All that may be required is to modify your work plans or adjust the milestones for the project. If your planning was done properly and the problem was identified early enough, it is unlikely that there will be serious consequences. However, whatever the nature of the divergence, it is important to maintain the momentum of the project and to take decisive action, at the same time being careful not to take hasty or ill-considered decisions. Avoid putting the project on hold, unless absolutely necessary, as this will cause your team to lose motivation and enthusiasm, and make them feel you are 'dithering'. Also, be sure to explain exactly what is being done and the reason for any delays you have been forced to agree on.

In addition, emphasize that having to take corrective action does not imply failure. It is natural for any system to be subject to stresses and variants, and many mechanical ones have devices built into them which continually bring them into line with the original course set, like an automatic pilot. Projects are no exception. What matters is that you anticipate it will happen, and deal with it when it does.

Stage 5

Completing the project

To complete the project, all the various threads of activity must be drawn together to ensure that:

- aims and objectives have been met
- project deliverables have been produced to schedule and to the quality standards agreed
- criteria and procedures laid down by sponsoring and funding agencies have been adhered to
- information has been collected to enable an evaluation of the project to be carried out
- any dissemination activities have been planned and are being undertaken.

This is not the end of the project as a whole; that comes after the evaluation has been carried out, plus any dissemination of the project's outcomes and findings. Rather it is the end of the *activity* stage which led to the project deliverables or products – now there will be time to pause and look over what has been achieved and consider whether it was successful.

Monitoring of progress in the implementation stage should have kept the project on course and ensured that any deviations or slippages were noted and remedial action taken. If this has worked effectively, the final deadline should not pose any real problems or present any difficulties.

Nevertheless, the final stages of a project can often be traumatic. For one thing, however carefully you pace yourself and your team and try to allow plenty of time for administration, there are usually far more forms and reports to complete than you envisaged. Where a project has received funding from an external source such as a European Union programme, the funding agency may require complicated and time-consuming final reports and returns to be made at the end of the project. At the outset, there may have been no clear indication of what would be required at project conclusion, and you may have under-estimated the time needed for filling in returns. Consequently, the last couple of weeks of a project's life often see the project team rushing around frantically trying to collect all the information required and process it by the deadline imposed.

Prior to completion, all the information required for finally evalu-ating the success of the project and the validity of its outcomes must be collected and processed.

Stage 6

Disseminating and evaluating the project

Evaluation is basically the process of making judgements about the success of the project. This is a twofold exercise: one aspect to be examined is the organization, implementation and management of the project itself, and the other is the quality of the project's outcomes and products.

Formative evaluation has, in effect, been on-going throughout the life of the project. During the implementation stage, performance was monitored and reviewed continually so that judgements were made about standards of achievement, which were in turn fed back into the project to effect improvements.

A previous section included information on the on-going monitoring and evaluation which took place during implementation. This section deals mainly with the final evaluation which takes place at the end of the project. Usually, the form this will take will have been identified and agreed at the planning stage, so that you will have been working towards it for some time. As you completed each milestone or workpackage, it was assessed against its original, proposed achievements, and the evaluation noted and fed back into the project cycle.

Where the project was concerned with producing or developing something, the model should be tested in its prototype state. This 'beta testing' can be done by using samples of people who would be typical users or beneficiaries of the product in its final form. Their views and experiences should be taken into account when carrying out final modifications and improvements to the product, prior to its final evaluation.

During the final evaluation stage, all of the formative assessments made by yourself and the team will be drawn together and combined with evaluations from other sources, and a summative evaluation made of the project as a whole. This will enable you and the team to decide how well you met your original objectives and how successful your project has been. It will also provide useful information to feed back into the organizations involved and to inform the work of other or future project teams.

Dissemination

Something which you will probably also want to do at the end of the project is to disseminate its outcomes. This task may be imposed upon you by funding agencies, but if not, do try to build it in anyway. If your project outcomes are not shared as widely as possible, the useful work you did is confined to a small field, and is of no benefit to others in the wider service.

Dissemination is also something you can build into the evaluation process, and the two can be readily combined. For example, you could use a dissemination conference to present the work you have done to a selected audience, and then enlist their help in evaluating it. You could ask delegates to complete a questionnaire or feedback sheet during the course of the event, or post it back afterwards, or ask them to volunteer to participate in some follow-up interviews.

At the planning stage, you gave some thought to your dissemination strategy and asked the questions *why, what, how, when* and *who.* These questions can help to shape the broad outlines of a dissemination plan, and as suggested earlier, dissemination can be on-going rather than simply seen as an add-on at the end of the project.

Asking the question '*why?*' helps you to focus on the heart of the dissemination. What is the point of doing it? Is your work of any value to anyone else, or is it so narrowly-based and specific that it is of interest only within your own organization (this is most unlikely). *What* are you disseminating? To what degree are you going to share your work; will you restrict it to project outcomes, with an explanation of the background and methodology, or are you going to share knowledge and information right through the lifespan of the project? If you have produced something which is commercially viable, how do you get this across? One way will obviously be to stress the quality standards built into the work, and if it has a technological aspect, you need to be able to show that it is state of the art.

How is one of the easier questions. The methods and channels you use will be largely dictated by the context in which the project operates and the audience it concerns. There is no point paying a computer wizard (a 'Webmaster') to create a page for you on the World Wide Web, if your target audience only has access to the printed page. There are various channels of communication which can be activated for dissemination purposes. Some of these may already have been used during the lifespan of the project so that dissemination is a continuous process – which relates to the question, *when?* For example, you might have produced regular bulletins or newsletters about your project and the last one of these would sum up the project's achievements as a whole, and perhaps invite contributions to the final evaluation. Aim for methods of dissemination that are effective, whether or not they are high-tech.

Who is another easy question in terms of targeting your dissemination. It is fairly straightforward to decide who to send information to, which staff to invite to conferences and meetings, and so on. But sending information out is one thing, and making sure it gets to the right people and is read by them is another. If your dissemination conference looks high-profile, you may find that your invited audience is overruled by their managers, who attend instead. Not high-profile enough, and the converse will happen. Try to send postal information to named individuals, if possible, and if there is an opportunity to make telephone contact as well, all the better.

A word of warning to those involved in transnational dissemination: attitudes in different countries are simply not the same. For example, some are more open to new technologies than others. Some want to spend a lot of time on the detail of processes and methodologies, whilst others want to examine the outcomes in detail and discuss their possible implications. Be prepared to take account of these cultural differences and try to appreciate the diversity of approach and breadth of experience they represent: getting impatient or patronizing, feeling superior (and even worse, sometimes showing it!) is no way to get the best out of your partners.

Evaluation – cast the net wide

Don't rely on one source or a single perspective for an evaluation of your work. Try to get a variety of feedback, and focus particularly on those people at whom your project is aimed. There is, of course, no one typical evaluation plan; they are as individual as projects are themselves. However, as a rough guide, an evaluation might involve the following:

- the **project team**
- an **external evaluator** such as a consultant
- **stakeholders** or **sponsors** or their representatives
- a sample of **clients** or people who could benefit from what the project has produced
- a sample of **staff** who might use the product as part of their work
- people who have been contacted via the **dissemination programme.**

Each of these groups would evaluate the project from their own point of view, reflecting their own particular concerns and priorities. The evaluation exercise therefore needs to be carefully structured and firmly directed, whilst not being so rigid that the responses received are of limited use.

The **project team** obviously know their project inside out. They are intimately acquainted with every facet of it and have detailed knowledge of everything that has happened during its lifespan. They have a valuable and unique part to play in evaluating its achievement. They have also had time to develop the kind of relationship that enables supportive self and team assessment. All the work put in during project planning and implementation to build the team's confidence and their ability to deal with criticism should now pay off. If good working relationships have been initiated and nurtured, it should be possible by now for colleagues to be open and honest with each other, working within an atmosphere of mutual trust.

However, they also suffer from a drawback which derives from their unique role and perspective – they are too involved with the project to be sure of being unbiased and objective in their assessments. This is not least because the success of project outcomes is closely linked with their own performance, and however honest they may want to be about that, they will simply be unable to step outside their own perception. This is why an external input is required.

The **external evaluator** has an extremely valuable part to play but, again, is to be regarded as a component part of any evaluation system rather than its totality. In some circumstances, sponsors or funding bodies may introduce a monitor or evaluator of their own, and this is discussed in the next point. The external evaluator considered in this point is one who is recruited and appointed by the organization managing the project, and works with the project manager.

When planning how evaluation will be managed, the role and remit of external consultants should be made clear, with a role specification being produced at an early stage as advised in the section on **Planning the project**. If they are being required to scrutinize any particular aspect in depth, this should be outlined in the specification.

The external evaluators should be introduced as soon as possible to the project team, who should be encouraged to think of them as 'critical friends'.

Evaluators need to have in-depth knowledge of the project and also to have a good understanding of the context in which it operates. They will want to visit sites and speak to key staff, and also to have access to documentation and records.

Stakeholders or **sponsors** may have their own evaluation agenda which might focus on the aspects of the project with which they are particularly concerned. For example, in the case of European projects receiving funding from the European Union, and operating trans-nationally, the funding agency will want to have evidence of the 'value added' by this international dimension. They will also want a clear description of how this is to be measured, in your evaluation plan.

Clients may sometimes also be seen as **beneficiaries**, in the sense of people who are deriving benefit from the project or its outcomes. If you intend to involve the beneficiaries of your project in the evaluation system, they should be briefed on this as soon as possible and care should be taken to ensure that they thoroughly understand the nature and purpose of the exercise. If their views are to have any real value, the project team must avoid the temptation to involve those select few who are known to be 'satisfied customers'.

Where projects will have products that will be used by **staff**, their feedback on the value of these outcomes is obviously essential. In the case of a piece of research or developmental work resulting in a new technique or piece of equipment, they will be the ones having to make the thing work. They will quite rightly complain if they have the final product imposed on them when it is fully-formed and unalterable, so make sure that they are involved in both formative and summative evaluation, as described earlier.

The **dissemination programme** has been discussed already. If your programme was ongoing (e.g. via regular newsletters, plus perhaps a dissemination conference) those people involved have been in the position of interested observers. Gaining feedback from a sample of them can provide valuable, broader perspectives on the project and its outcomes.

What are you evaluating?

Whoever you involve, the primary rule is to be clear about what you are evaluating. It is easy at this stage to get so bogged down in the minute detail of your project that you lose sight of what you were aiming to achieve in the first place. Refresh your memory by going back to the original aims and objectives, and the outcomes you identified at the start. You are now trying to decide if your project has done its job. Have you achieved your goal? And how well have you achieved it?

In order to do this, you need to identify the object or thing you aimed to produce and its characteristics. You did this at the beginning of the project, during the planning stage, but since then may have modified your project outcomes as your work proceeded. Now you must 'revisit' them, together with the characteristics you defined for them. For example, many projects are concerned with producing something innovatory. If you proposed to do this, you will have examined what 'innovatory' meant during planning. You will also have agreed how you would measure or assess this. Now you need to find out whether you really have produced something new, as well as assessing the value or usefulness of your product.

This may not be a concrete, physical object, but may be some form of new practice or a model approach capable of transfer elsewhere. When you planned the project, you spent a lot of time on quality control mechanisms, including defining success criteria, creating a monitoring system and planning your evaluation strategy. You used these during the lifespan of the project to keep your work on course and ensure that you maintained the standards deemed appropriate. Now is the time to take a step back and look at the project from a distance. It might be helpful to produce a final evaluation checklist to help you to look at the project as a whole (an example is provided in the **Toolkit**). This is why using 'outsiders' can be so valuable at this stage, as they are likely to be able to take an objective view. By this time, you and your team may be finding it very difficult to be objective, especially as you may have invested a lot in the project and may be unwilling to perceive it as a failure in any way. Don't worry about this, it is perfectly normal. Recognize it and work *with* it, rather than trying to deny how you feel.

Appendix 1

Writing a project proposal

Producing a written proposal is usually an early requirement in any project, and the complexity of this is determined by the funding or sponsoring agency. If external funding or grant aid is being sought, the agency holding the funds will often dictate the component parts of the proposal and may issue a form to be completed by a certain deadline.

As a rough guide, however, there tend to be certain information requirements which are common to all proposals. Much of these are covered in the main section, but this appendix deals with some aspects in more detail.

Aims and objectives of the project

The overall **aim** of your project is usually its *purpose* in general terms, that is, what it intends to achieve or accomplish. The **objectives** are more specific than this and are broken down into discrete and more detailed actions. For example:

Aim

- To improve the experience of people using the out-patient facilities of the Ophthalmic Unit of Moorland View Hospital.

Objectives

- Identify areas of dissatisfaction with the current service, in consultation with patients and staff, and identify ways of eliminating these.

- Gather information on best practice in similar units and explore how this could be integrated into Moorland View's practice.

- Agree quality standards for the unit in agreed areas (e.g. waiting time, facilities available whilst waiting, briefing of patients by clinical staff, explanations about the system in use, documentary information available to patients, etc.).

- Formulate and agree procedures to implement improvements.

- Assess the impact of improvements, and evaluate the benefits.

- Disseminate the outcomes to other units of the hospital.

Indicators of success

Also sometimes known as **achievement indicators**. These are the quantifiable changes which have come about as a result of your project. They are generally things which can be measured and proved, for example, in relation to numbers of people, amounts of time and so on. If you are asked to provide these at proposal stage, make sure that the ones you set yourself are achievable!

A difficulty with indicators of success is that they may not be very useful for measuring fine differences or for measuring qualitative changes in certain circumstances. They need some careful thought and a regard for the context in which the project will operate. For example, it would be no use simply identifying an indicator of success at the Moorview eye unit such as 'fewer complaints about waiting time'. There may be no complaints about waiting time because people just put up with it and associate NHS treatment with long waits. Better indicators could be things like reductions in the actual lengths of time waited, and patient perception that there has been improvement (for instance, via data gained from a survey).

Project outcomes or deliverables

These are the things which the project will actually *produce* by the end of its lifespan. They may include new or additional knowledge, innovative systems or ways of doing things, improvements in expertise and skill, or material benefits like a more prosperous or revitalized economy, a more efficient service or a pleasanter working environment. Whatever they are, they should be things which actually make a difference in some way – otherwise the project has been a waste of time. They will usually be *recorded*, often by a project report. External funding, especially from public sources, is usually dependent upon the outcomes of projects being shared widely so that service-users derive maximum benefit from them. Funding agencies often require applications to show how the outcomes of projects will be *disseminated*. In some cases, where a new product is being developed, funding agencies may want to know that it will be commercially viable after the project funding has been exhausted.

Costings

The most expensive element in a project is usually staff time. This means that it is usually impossible to accurately estimate costs until the timescale of the project has been worked out, and its staffing needs identified.

Project leaders or initiators are always under pressure to produce costings and an overall budget for their projects, for obvious reasons. Often the project is being funded under a programme such as those established by the European Union, perhaps for research and development, or for training. Sponsors and funding agencies have global budgets to allocate for their programmes and are concerned not to over or underspend. They are likely to require project leaders to provide information on exact costings at the application stage of externally-funded projects (at this point, there is often no way of paying for work to be undertaken on the project and staff are having to do it alongside their existing workloads).

Many funding agencies will provide headings under which costs must be broken down, and will also provide detailed guidelines on what costs are 'allowable', in other words, eligible to be included in the budget for the project. Most agencies will provide only part-funding for projects and expect the organization proposing the work to contribute to it themselves. Sometimes this contribution can be in kind rather than in cash, for example, office space and equipment. Sometimes the costs of depreciation of equipment can be taken into account, and a formula may be provided for this. In most cases, funding agencies will not allow their money to be used to make capital purchases (e.g. new computers or office furniture) but may permit the cost of hiring or leasing to be included in the allowable costs.

If your project is likely to have costs which are not eligible under the rules of the programme concerned, you may need to identify these separately on your budget and make provision for them out of your own organization's budgets. You will then need to make this clear both at the application stage and at the end of your project, to avoid any confusion and to reassure the external funding agency that you are adhering to their rules.

Keeping accurate records of all costs and transactions is extremely important. Whoever handles the finance side of your project should be fully briefed about the rules applying to project funding, and the project leader or manager should make periodic checks on financial records to make sure they are in order and conform to the requirements of the funding body. Failure to do this could lead to charges of fraud, and there have been several cases where projects have been stopped overnight after a monitoring visit from the external funder, and all monies withdrawn. In such cases, the funding agency may also claim back the funding already given, on the grounds that it was not spent properly.

If your funding agency does not provide a budget structure, or if you are lucky enough to have an internally-funded project, you may need to devise your own budget headings, in consultation with your finance officer. Some typical headings are:

- **Human resources**. This includes all staffing for your project, plus any external consultants or temporary staff. Your funding agency may require you to specify salary costs for different levels of staff, plus their other costs such as national insurance contributions, etc. Some programmes specifically exclude the use of external consultants, but perversely may allow you to 'buy in' technical advice!

Your staffing costs (and others, too) will increase if your project runs for more than one year, as your staff will probably receive pay increases, and these should be incorporated.

- **Equipment**. For large items, this might be the cost of buying, hiring or leasing new equipment or it might be the depreciation costs of existing equipment. Small items such as computer disks, books, printer ribbons, paper and so on can be regarded as 'consumables' because they will be used up at the end of the project.

- **Travel and subsistence**. This will have to be a broad estimate, with staff using the usual mileage rate for your organization. Try to err on the side of generosity; it is easy to underestimate the amount of travelling you may need to do, especially if several sites are involved in the project. For long distance travel (for example, in the case of international or EU projects) you will need to identify *how many* meetings will take place, *where* and *which staff* will attend them, before you can calculate the cost. Even if you are linked by email and fax, there is no substitute for personal meetings and you are bound to need a few.

- **Telephone, fax and other running costs**. These may need to be charged proportionately to your project, if you are sharing them with others in your organization (keeping a fax log may be one way to record use of this). Again, make a generous estimate at the costings stage, based upon the number of people involved in your project and where they are based. The communications strategies you use in your project will inevitably have cost implications, for example, postage costs may be high if you are doing a lot of project dissemination by news bulletin. Ditto your photocopying or printing charges. You may also need to include other office running costs such as heat and light, security, caretaking and cleaning services costs, etc.

- **Training and staff development**. This should include the costs of any internally-organized training workshops in support of the project, such as record-keeping, or bought-in training such as language learning. These can be identified fairly easily in advance and costed out.

- **Contingencies**. These will inevitably arise, however carefully you plan. Many of the things which arise during your project's lifespan will be outside your control. Other occurrences may have been unforeseen, simply due to human error. There is no need for recriminations and panic if you set up a contingency fund (say, at 5–10% of your project budget) to allow for this. Ensure that your funding agency or sponsor knows what you plan and will also allow you to vire money from the contingency fund into any other category. If this is the case, you can top up any overspend elsewhere in your budget from the contingency fund. Keep the amount relatively small – 10% or below – so that if it is never used, you are not returning an embarrassing amount to your sponsor.

Don't forget that all your costs are subject to inflation, and that if your project has a long lifespan, you need to increase your estimated costs proportionally from one year to the next.

Dissemination

Only in very rare cases is there no value in disseminating the results of a project. Certainly, all those which qualify for external funding will have transferable outcomes and will need to have a dissemination strategy built in, either as part of or prior to, the final evaluation. The methods used for dissemination will depend upon the nature of the project and its outcomes and could include newsletters, items on the World Wide Web, conferences or seminars, etc.

Monitoring and evaluation

Funding agencies are keen to ensure that they are getting value for money and a quality result, so they usually want to know about your monitoring and evaluation systems at the application stage. It may not be necessary to provide detailed information and you may simply be required to outline the methods you would use. You need to stress that you will be monitoring throughout, and undertaking formative evaluations which will be fed back into the implementation process, not simply leaving evaluation until the end of the project.

Exploitation and commercial viability

This is important for those research and development projects which aim to create an end product that will be able to stand on its own after project funding has run out. You may be required to produce an exploitation plan which shows that your product will be viable, perhaps as a purely commercial proposition if this is appropriate. For many projects, this may simply be a matter of working with a commercial company who will produce and market your product under licence, but the way in which this would be organized should be described in the proposal. The question of intellectual property must also be clarified; in other words, who owns the research that will be done during the project and the outcomes which will result from it.

Appendix 2

Total Quality Management (TQM)

It is generally accepted that the concept of Total Quality originated in Japan, as a result of the impact of approaches introduced to the Japanese by American 'quality gurus' in the context of post-war reconstruction, and most notably by Dr W. Edwards Deming. It began as a philosophy developed for the manufacturing industry, but has since found its way into the service sector and has been adapted for use in health, education and local government services of all kinds.

The idea of the possibility of Total Quality and the belief that it could be managed as a process was successful in the Japanese context because it requires commitment, and the Japanese culture of company loyalty ensured an ideal environment for such ideas to develop, once accepted by top management.

TQM is seen as an approach in which the commitment of top management is essential. Everyone in the company or organization is responsible for ensuring quality, but the lead comes down from the top. Managers are then responsible for inducting the workforce into the principles of TQM and employees must be aware of the basic concepts behind it, and sufficiently motivated to make them work.

The underlying principle is that errors and mistakes are preventable and that it is possible to produce goods which are fault-free. It is also the premise of TQM that processes and products can be continually improved.

TQM usually requires organizational change, which can be resisted if commitment is not secured from the start. First, it relies upon the collection and manipulation of data in an objective way. Information should be collected on current working practices and processes, on organizational structures and their interaction, on failure rates or the number of times targets are not met, etc. However, many organizations feel they know their markets and products, not to mention their own operational processes, very well, and are resistant to the collection of information on them.

Also, TQM operates on the principle that there are two kinds of relationship in organizations, 'suppliers' and 'customers'. Some of these may be so quite literally, but others are only occupying the relationship of customers or suppliers *internally*. Organizations consist of a network of staff interacting as customers and suppliers of services. For instance, a clerical assistant is supplying a service to another officer, who is in turn his/her customer. This clarification of internal customer relationships is crucial to the success of the system. However, it can uncover dependencies which are unwelcome revelations to those in positions of authority.

At the end of the chain are the *external* customers and suppliers. Again, TQM is about developing effective relationships based on mutual understanding between organizations and their customers, and those who supply them with goods and services. The idea is that an organization works with its suppliers to educate them and help them understand exactly what is required so that the supplier can then provide the appropriate goods or services more efficiently. In certain situations, it may be possible for requirements to be anticipated or exceeded.

The same goes for customers, that is, the organization needs to ensure that it understands the needs and preferences of its customers and the existing degree of customer satisfaction.

In addition, TQM focuses the organization's attention upon the costs of poor quality, not just in monetary terms but in staff motivation and other areas.

The concept of continuous or never-ending improvement is also seen as something requiring organizational change. It should not be imposed upon the workforce, driving them to work under greater pressure and making impossible demands, but as a challenge which energizes staff and motivates them, and as something in which they are fully involved. Once targets have been met, new ones can be designated, and the organization can not only gain a competitive edge but maintain it, keeping ahead of others in the field.

Deming's TQM system was based upon 14 points, one of which – 'Take action to accomplish the transformation' – relies upon a process known as the 'PDCA cycle', which stands for 'Plan, Do, Check, Act'. This was originally known as 'The Shewhart Cycle' because it was invented by a statistician of that name, and modified in turn by Deming.

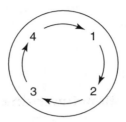

Figure 1 The PDCA Cycle

Step 1 is to study a process and decide how it might be improved, and create a **plan** before taking any action. **Step 2** involves **doing** the agreed action, or making the necessary changes. **Step 3** is the observation stage when the Quality Team check the effects of their action. **Step 4** involves studying the results of the action and may require the test to be repeated before it can be acted upon. The cycle is repeated in the future with knowledge and experience being accumulated and an upward spiral of continuous improvement being created.

In conclusion, the basic principles of TQM can be summarized as follows:

• Understand and develop the customer relationships of the organization.
• Make a commitment to continuous improvement.
• Understand and control your organization's working processes.
• Plan to prevent faults rather than detecting and weeding them out.
• Involve all staff in preventative action.
• Promote commitment from all staff, starting with management, to the TQM process.

Appendix 3

Benchmarking

The word 'benchmarking' is borrowed from land surveying, where a point selected as a base for surveys, and cut into rock or marked in some way, is called a benchmark. Within the Quality movement, the term is used for the practice of measuring and comparing aspects of your organization with other organizations to define standards of performance. The technique began to be widely used after it was adopted by Rank Xerox in 1979. American managers in Rank Xerox plants were sent to study the working practices of their Japanese counterparts and compare performance. Where improvements in performance and standards were identified, the managers were encouraged to scrutinize how these had come about and assess the potential for transfer of good practice.

Within the manufacturing industry, benchmarking is now an accepted procedure which many companies undertake as a matter of course. Organizations within a benchmarking partnership or network will usually adopt a structured approach, often selecting a single aspect of working practice as the focus for each exercise. The idea is to identify the best practice and adopt it, or even to improve upon it, modifying as necessary.

Aspects to be compared could include:

- customer satisfaction
- internal communications
- communication with service-users
- costs

- methods and practices used in different sections of the organization
- staff training and development
- staffing structures.

Where organizations are not in direct competition, it is possible to work together fairly openly and co-operate without constraint. Within the public sector, this tends to be the case even where organizations are involved in the same type of work. In the private sector, competing companies may sometimes undertake 'covert' benchmarking, e.g. buying the competitor's product, stripping it down and studying it, or carrying out a survey of their customers.

Various methods are used for benchmarking exercises, including:

- product or service examination, which can involve dismantling and technical data collection
- surveys of staff or customers
- analysis of published material, such as information leaflets, annual reports
- using consultants as assessors
- exchange visits between staff doing similar jobs
- study visits or joint workshops.

As with many other techniques, it is important to avoid the adoption of an over-simplistic approach, and to view organizations holistically rather than piecemeal. A benchmarking exercise on staffing ratios for support staff which relies solely on statistics may suggest that one organization is over-staffed in that area. However, it may then be necessary to identify how staff are being defined, what roles they undertake and how they contribute to organizational effectiveness – are there fewer managers, say, because they are better supported? Getting an overall view of the organization before studying a single aspect, so that the benchmarking exercise is viewed in context, would avoid such simplistic misconceptions.

Appendix 4

The PRINCE project management system

The PRINCE project management system was developed for use by Government departments, and is now widely used in a variety of contexts, though initially it was intended as an IT-related methodology. It is quite complex and has many specific component parts, and is itself the subject of several bulky manuals and guides. It is beyond the scope of this Appendix to do more than simply summarize the main features of the system; for more detail, readers should consult one of the publications mentioned at the end of this section.

PRINCE claims to differ from other project management techniques by focusing on the products to be produced by the project rather than its activities. (In fact, this is rather unfair as many modern project management systems concentrate equally on processes and deliverables rather than being preoccupied by methods, as the advocates of PRINCE suggest.)

The planning process begins with the clarification of the central goal, and the identification of all anticipated products of the project. Once this has been done and a common understanding reached between those involved, the activities necessary to achieve these products are identified. The focus is always on the goal rather than the means of achieving it, on products rather than methods.

The system involves the use of three techniques, Product Breakdown Structures, Product Flow Diagrams and Product Descriptions, which are regarded as being interdependent.

Product Breakdown Structures (PBS) identify all the products which will result from the project. A product is defined as 'an object that will be delivered by the project which can be seen, felt and measured. People . . . can be considered to be products, if their state is to be changed, for example, "Trained Users" are a valid project product'.

(From The PRINCE Training Pack, November 1991, Duhig Berry Ltd.)

The main categories of product are:

- Management products – which enable effective project management, e.g. plans, job descriptions.
- Technical products – which will exist after the project has ended, to maintain and enhance systems, e.g. user manuals, programs.
- Quality products – which ensure the quality of systems and outputs, e.g. product descriptions, reports.
- External products – which are necessary for the success of the project but may already exist or are outside its scope, e.g. company manuals, products of other, associated projects.

The Product Breakdown Structure requires the technical products to be defined first, then the management products, then the quality products. The PBS is refined after the Product Flow Diagram has been produced to include any more products which have been identified as part of that process. The PBS is then broken down into stages, which in turn are refined.

Product Flow Diagrams describe the logical sequence for developing the products identified via the PBS, together with the 'dependencies' identified. They must not be allowed to become too complicated or planners will lose sight of the products and become preoccupied with the activities and methods.

Product Descriptions describe each of the products identified on the PBS and have the following components:

- the **purpose** of the product and why it is to be produced
- its **composition**, in line with the PBS
- the **form** it will take
- its **derivation** and the sources from which it originated
- the **quality criteria** by which it will be measured
- the **quality control method** used for checking the product against the quality criteria.

PRINCE places considerable emphasis on the planning stage of projects and outlines in detail the functions of planning. Two types of plan are identified. The Activity Plan is usually expressed as a bar chart, and shows how activities are spread across timescales. The Resource Plan is expressed as a table and identifies the resources required to support the Activity Plan, and includes staffing elements, equipment and software and the costs of each.

In addition, there should be a Graphical Summary plotting the deliverables, timescales and expenditure for the project. Stage Plans are produced to control each stage of the project, and ensure that one stage is properly completed before another is begun.

The **control** of projects is also a major concern of PRINCE, with the focus being upon measuring and monitoring. The guidance on this indicates that a Project Board should be established involving senior management and representing the three interests of the project, namely the User, the Technical (IT) and the Business (that is, value for money) interests. A Project Assurance Team should then be appointed consisting of three Co-ordinators representing and responsible for the three interests, and these individuals will undertake the monitoring role, remaining independent of the day-to-day operation of the project. PRINCE lays down detailed guidance on the subsequent monitoring process and the criteria for measuring achievement, and defines the major 'control points'

PRINCE similarly lays down an **organizational** structure with detailed specifications for the role of key staff and teams.

Reading

A complete set of PRINCE documentation is available from:

The Publications Manager, National Computing Centre Ltd, Oxford Road, Manchester M1 7ED.

Appendix 5

Systems of quality standards – BS 5750, ISO 9000 and EN 29000

The universal concern with quality in the world of industry and commerce has given rise to the development of certificated systems of quality standards.

In the UK, the quality standard known as BS 5750 was first published in 1979. Other national standards were devised and introduced in countries elsewhere, some of them based on BS 5750, and this led to the International Organization for Standardization (ISO) developing an international standard in order to rationalize matters. Work began in 1983, but it was not until 1987 that a series of five standards was published as ISO 9000.

ISO 9000 is largely based on BS 5750, tempered by several years of usage and taking into account the requirements of an international target audience. In Europe, the standard had been adopted as EN 29000.

All of this might sound confusing to those who are unfamiliar with this area. To clarify then, the BS 5750 series is the British standard, the ISO 9000 is the international series of standards, and the EN 29000 is the European series. These systems provide manufacturers and suppliers with the requirements for a quality system. The principles of the systems are intended to be applicable to any company, however large or small, and identify basic procedures and criteria for quality products and systems.

Section 2

The Project Management Toolkit

Some of the tools for doing the job

Brainstorming

As the name of this tool suggests, it is intended to help with generating ideas. Each person has a store of experience and information unique to himself or herself, but this often needs to be triggered in order for it to be released. This technique provides the trigger by encouraging people to think laterally and creatively.

How to do it

1. Explain the technique

Tell the group what brainstorming is and get their commitment to using it. Identify the purpose of the session and agree a statement with the group about this, so that it can provide a focus. Write it out and stick it on the wall (or on a whiteboard) and have a flipchart on hand to note down ideas. Post-it notes can be particularly useful.

2. Outline the rules

Get everyone to agree to a set of rules. These are:

Rule 1. All ideas offered will be noted down, however 'off the wall' they may initially appear.

Rule 2. There is to be no discussion of ideas whilst brainstorming is in session, apart from any necessary clarification.

Rule 3. Repetition is allowed – there is to be no ruling out of ideas at this stage.

Rule 4. No questions are allowed (other than to clarify what an idea means).

3. Run the session

Make sure someone (yourself?) acts as leader and ensures that the rules are not broken.

Use a framework to encourage the freeflow of ideas such as one (or a combination) of these:

Random contributions – if people are likely to work well as a group, simply invite ideas from anyone.

Individual contributions – if people are shy, or unsure about the technique, give them five minutes to write ideas down in silence, then share them with the group.

Taking it in turns – arrange the group in a circle or horseshoe and invite an idea from each, allowing people to say 'pass' if they want to.

If ideas run out, try suggesting something bizarre or deliberately funny to get things going again.

List all the ideas on flipchart paper and put them up around the walls of the room, dividing them up into categories.

4. Evaluate the ideas

(This process will differ according to the focus of the brainstorming session.)

Go through all the ideas with the group and:

eliminate those which everyone agrees are non-starters;

select viable ones from the list and discuss and develop them, with a view to agreeing priorities which will then be built into your plan of action.

Note: it can be useful to keep the flipcharts after the session is completed, as the ideas on them may be useful in the future.

Toolkit sheet 2

Project team skills specification

Project Requirement	Skills/expertise needed	Person/grade to be involved
Knowledge about . . .		
Experience of . . .		

Skills in . . .		
Personal qualities/ other attributes . . .		

Skills for project management

A self-assessment checklist

Put a tick or cross in the box to indicate whether you have the skills or experience identified.

Use the ticks to identify where you already have the skill or experience, and use the space below to note down any specific details which might be useful.

Use the crosses to identify your areas of weakness. Decide if you need any training in these areas or whether you can work on a weakness in other ways, or develop strategies for minimising it. You can make notes about this in the space below.

Use the extra space at the end to add any special additional skills needed by your own project.

(If a particular point does not apply to your project and cannot be addressed at present, delete it, but also note it for your own staff development needs in the future.)

☐ I am an efficient organizer and have organized events or activities before which have run smoothly

☐ My memory is good and I never forget anything important

☐ I make sure that everything I do is to the highest quality that circumstances allow

☐ I am reliable and always punctual for business meetings

☐ I am good at motivating people and can always get them fired up with enthusiasm about an idea

☐ My presentational skills are good and I know how to speak effectively in public

☐ I am good at managing meetings and interacting with people

☐ I can communicate well on paper and present issues and facts succinctly and clearly

☐ I have experience in writing reports, agendas and other routine business communications

☐ I have worked within time constraints and am good at keeping to schedule

☐ I can work with other people in a team setting and have good negotiating skills

☐ I have experience and knowledge of financial management and know how to produce and work within a budget

☐ I know how to access information and set up information systems

☐ I have a basic grounding in IT skills and no fear of computers

☐ I have experience of record-keeping and know about audit procedures

☐ I stay calm under pressure and never panic if there is a crisis

☐ I understand how to set measurable objectives and monitor these

☐ I know how to measure and evaluate achievement against stated objectives and outcomes

☐ I am familiar with my organization's development plan/corporate plan and our mission statement

☐ I have researched into other business/international cultures/perspectives

☐ I am familiar with international time zones/systems

☐ I can communicate with my international partners in their language

Project manager – roles and responsibilities

- Identify clear aims and objectives for the project.
- Define roles and responsibilities of partners and staff.
- Ensure all documentation is completed accurately, appropriately and to deadlines, including all reports and plans.
- Agree budgets and ensure adequate financial management and monitoring procedures.
- Manage team meetings and contribute to Steering Group meetings
- Manage and supervise all project staff, monitoring their performance.
- Ensure close communication and collaboration with partners.
- Maintain communication with project consultants and supervise their input.
- Liaise with other relevant projects and teams and ensure that the project benefits from other R & D findings as appropriate.
- Report regularly to the Departmental Director and comply with procedures ensuring accountability.

Project planning
techniques – taskboarding

This is a simple technique and requires little more equipment than a flip chart and pens, pencil, rubber and a couple of pads of the largest size of Post-it notes or similar self-adhesive notelets.

To work at its best, this is a technique that requires some initial planning to have been done, so that you have some idea of the key stages of your project. (This was undertaken in Section 1, using a method like brainstorming, for instance.)

Session 1

Working as a team, list the key stages you have identified in preparatory planning, reviewing the list as you go along. You may wish to add stages or break some down further as you think about them.

Then write down the title of every key stage on a notelet, using the top half only. Stick them in any order on one wall or table surface. Designate another wall or area as the 'taskboard'. (If you are away from the office in another venue, use a large board or a series of flip chart pages which you can take away with you.)

The key stages might include items like:

- carry out survey of clients
- obtain IT equipment
- submit bid for funding
- train staff to use software.

Now decide as a group which one of your key stages comes first. (This may prove to be quite difficult, but don't worry too much if you get it wrong; as the session progresses, you will be able to reassess your first decision and simply move the notelets around.) Move this notelet to the top of the planning area. Work through the lifespan of your project, moving notelets across to the taskboard as you decide where they belong in the timescale. Do this by having one member of the group ask the others questions after each one is placed, such as:

'have we got everything we need in order to complete all the tasks in this stage?' – which will enable you to check that everything is in place to support the tasks in that stage so that you can go on to the next. (You will almost certainly find on occasions that something has been overlooked or omitted, or put in at the wrong stage.)
'what can we do now that this stage is in place?'
'what do we need to do next?'

By the end of this first session, you will have a logical representation of the project in key stages. You might like to take a break at this point, perhaps for a day or more, in order to have some time for reflection. The taskboard should be left in place so that people can revisit it and consider it further. You may also want to organize a review meeting before the next session, so that people can share their thoughts and ideas on any amendments or reorganization of the key stages, and the taskboard can be changed accordingly.

Session 2

In this session you will develop the taskboard so that each key stage will be confirmed in its place, be coded for other planning purposes and be given a duration in hours, days or weeks (depending upon the length and complexity of your project).

The coding should be by letter (A–Z) so that it does not become confused with timescales, which will, of course, be in numbers. Put the key stage code letter on the top left and the other (the time allotted) on the bottom right of the notelet. You now also need to work out how the key stages interrelate and are dependent upon each other. For example, staff cannot be trained on new software until it has been ordered, delivered and satisfactorily installed. This should have been identified as an earlier key stage and given a letter. You can make a note of each dependency on each notelet, too.

It will now look like Figure 2.

```
┌─────────────────────────────────────────┐
│ F                                        │
│                                          │
│ Train staff on new software              │
│                                          │
│                                          │
│ Dependent on: C          2 days          │
└─────────────────────────────────────────┘
```

Figure 2

You might want to stop now and have another break for reflection, before confirming the work done so far.

Session 3

Session 3 enables the team to confirm the taskboard or amend it following the period of reflection. Then all that remains is to transfer all the information from the notelets onto a printed taskboard which summarizes all the information and can be circulated to everyone involved.

The same technique can be used to break the tasks down further, into their component parts, if wished.

For simple projects which do not need to be broken down into milestones, the taskboard can take the place of a detailed implementation plan. For complex ones, it is a useful technique for taking planning on from the brainstorming stage to the point where each key stage can be scrutinised in detail and turned into a milestone.

Project milestone sheet

Milestone no.

Estimated start date:_____   Estimated completion date:_____

Actual start date:_____   Actual completion date:_____

Milestone value: £_____

Milestone tasks/ deliverables	Progressed by:	Start/finish	Monitored by:	On course/ slippage and remedial action:

Resources identification sheet

Task/activity	Staff	Services	Equipment/venue	Materials	Cost
Project team training on new software	1 IT trainer	Catering – lunch for 7	6 work stations 1 training room Flip chart OHP	6 training packs Printer Paper Diskettes	£160

Implementation plan

N.B. This is an extract from an actual Implementation Plan and is not complete. It relates to a project involving the production of a new staff training handbook.

Milestones and contract value	Objectives	Activities	Target date	Outcomes
Milestone 1 £800	Project initiation and start up	Set up project management, delivery and monitoring systems	End of September 1997	Documentation Flowchart Steering committee Management and admin. set up; also quality assurance Procedures
Milestone 2 £1500	Set up basis for collecting and using material for handbook	Develop project methodology into a design	Beginning of October 1997	Framework Selection specification and criteria produced, plus explanatory information
Milestone 3 £2500	Collect and produce material for handbook	Identify/invite contributions Collate and edit material Devise and consult on handbook format Prepare for dissemination	End of December 1997	Material to specification for all sections of handbook Format decided Publicity material agreed
Milestone 4 £2200	Prepare prototype handbook for limited field test	Complete editing Select testing partners, begin dissemination activities	End of January 1998	Handbook ready for field testing

Milestone 5 £2060	Pilot prototype	Issue prototype Monitor piloting Receive initial feedback Continue dissemination activities	Early March 1998	Evaluation of pilot test results

Cause and effect diagram

Using a Cause and Effect Diagram helps to unravel the causes or contributory factors which resulted in a particular effect. This effect may be a problem or mistake, in which case the CED can be used as the basis for the problem-solving exercise which:

- determines how the problem occurred
- provides insights into how it might have been avoided, which are valuable lessons for the present and future.

Conversely, it could be something positive or innovatory which your organization wants to duplicate or transfer. It can also be used as a tool for allocating tasks to individuals or groups.

This technique can be used by individuals, but is most often employed during group sessions or workshops. It can be a valuable tool for use in team building exercises.

Using cause and effect diagrams (Figure 3)

Write down the effect or problem in the box on the extreme right. Make this as detailed a statement or definition as possible, and make sure that team members agree on it. Then identify the main contributory factors or causes and divide these into categories. Assign each one to a branch or rib of the diagram, writing it into the box at the tip of the branch. Then work your way through the categories and list the causes or contributory factors in each one, writing them against the minor 'bones' of the fish. Make further subdivisions of categories if necessary. Take care not to confuse symptoms or outward

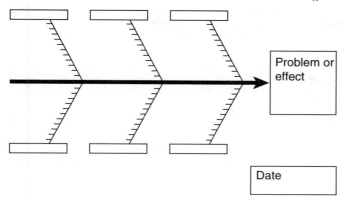

Figure 3 Cause and effect diagram

signs with the actual causes of the effect – the former are simply manifestations rather than actual causes.

Some basic rules should be followed, specifically:

- get your definition of the effect or problem right before starting, and make sure everyone agrees it is accurate
- go as far back as possible to discover the root of your causes
- be clear about statements made and don't use vague or woolly language
- be as specific as possible in describing events or issues.

Project monitoring and evaluation checklists

All project leaders and their teams need to devise their own individual monitoring tools, tailored to the requirements of their project. The following checklists are intended to serve merely as a broad template. Project leaders will need to produce 'customised' and more detailed checklists, focusing on aspects of their specific projects and the context in which they are set.

Checklist A   Project start-up

A1   Do all team members have a copy of the Project Implementation Plan, including a detailed set of project objectives with milestones?

A2   Have all team members been fully briefed as to their roles and responsibilities?

A3   Are systems in place for recording the use of project resources, including (as appropriate):

- logging of staff time
- logging of equipment and materials used
- logging of services used
  plus any other expenditure-related items?

A4   Are systems in place for recording any income generated by the project, if applicable?

A5   Do these systems conform with the quality standards or criteria established for them (and in conformity with the regulations of the funding/sponsoring organizations)?

Are they:

accurate
clear and legible
up-to-date
secure
confidential (if applicable)?

Checklist B   Project implementation

Project objectives and deliverables

B1   Are the original objectives proving to be appropriate and attainable? If not, why not, and how are they being adjusted?

B2   Are additional objectives and benefits being identified and agreed during the course of the project? How are they being recorded and monitored?

B3   Are the intended project deliverables proving to be realistic? If not, why not?

B4   Are team members being honestly objective about the progress and quality of deliverables and accurate in their assessment and recording of them?

B5   How quickly are areas of divergence being identified? Could this be improved?

B6   How well are corrective strategies working? Could they be improved?

Project timing and work schedules

B7   How are you ensuring that the project runs to the agreed timetable and that the milestones are met in time?

B8   Where amendments to work schedules are necessary, how are these being agreed and built in?

B9   How are they being communicated to project team members? Are they being recorded onto the Project Implementation Plan?

Documentation, record-keeping and financial management

B10   Is the range of documentation for the project meeting the quality standards identified?

B11 What systems are in place for maintaining records of:

- project plans?
- applications for funding?
- guidelines and regulations issued by funding agencies?
- internal regulations and codes of practice?
- staffing structures and roles/job descriptions?

B12 Can any improvements be identified and made to these systems and built in during implementation?

B13 Are all team members aware of financial regulations and adhering to them?

B14 Are all team members aware of record-keeping procedures and adhering to them?

B15 How are records being stored and maintained? Have any checks been made to sample the effectiveness of the system (e.g., a small-scale 'dummy' audit)?

B16 Can any improvements be identified and employed?

Other issues

B17 How is the project team ensuring that maximum use is made of transnational and external links? Are there any other useful spin-offs from any partnership arrangements made?

Checklist C   Final evaluation

Project outcomes or deliverables

C1   Have the intended outcomes of your project been achieved in terms of:

- the central object or product you aimed to deliver?
- the characteristics of the product as originally identified?

C2   If not, how do the outcomes differ from those originally proposed?

Project initiation and planning

C3   With hindsight, were the original aims, objectives and deliverables identified during the project planning stage viable and achievable?

C4 Was the planning for the project undertaken sufficiently thoroughly?

C5 Were the methods used effective?

C6 How might they have been improved?

Implementation

C7 Were the project deliverables actually achieved on time and to acceptable standards of quality? Which ones were not and why not?

C8 How well did your monitoring and formative evaluation system work? Could it have been improved?

C9 How well did the project team and other colleagues work together? Could this have been improved?

C10 Was the original timing for the project adequate in terms of:

- amount of time allowed for meeting objectives/producing deliverables?
- times of year when activities planned were proposed to take place?

Can any lessons for the future be learned from this?

C11 How well did your record-keeping and accounting system work? Could it have been better organized and maintained, and how?

C12 Does the project represent value for money? Looking at the final outcomes, could these have been achieved more economically?

C13 How well did any transnational links work? Do you feel you got all you could out of them? What problems were identified and how might these be overcome in any future project? What did you gain from having an international dimension?

Dissemination

C14 Do you think your dissemination strategy was effective? Could it have been improved?

Monitoring and evaluation

C15 How well do you feel your monitoring and evaluation system worked? Are you now able to effectively evaluate the overall success of the project? If not, why not?

Section 3

Project Management for Real

Real life examples of project work in the health care sector

Case Study 1

Developing a new undergraduate medical curriculum at Imperial College School of Medicine

Judy McKimm, MBA, MA(Ed), BA (Hons), Cert Ed
Assistant Director, Medical Education Unit, Imperial College of Science, Technology and Medicine, London

Origin of the project

The main aim of the project was to plan, design and implement a new medical undergraduate degree course, in accordance with the General Medical Council's recommendations on undergraduate clinical education embodied in *Tomorrow's Doctors* (1993).

The curriculum development project has been implemented alongside a much larger process, the merger of two undergraduate and two postgraduate Medical Schools into a new organization – Imperial College School of Medicine (ICSM). The processes of curriculum and organizational change cannot be considered as separate projects, and the management of the curriculum development project is essentially one of change management.

Changes in the external environment

All undergraduate medical curricula in the UK have to meet the requirements of the Higher Education Funding Council of England (HEFCE) and the Higher Education Quality Council (HEQC) as to quality of teaching provision, in common with all HE institutions. In addition, they must also meet the requirements of the General Medical Council (GMC), which 'licences' medical schools to train doctors.

Implicit in the training of doctors is the need to demonstrate to the Department of Health that undergraduate medical education and training reflects the needs of the NHS, which is a rapidly changing environment with increasing accountability. Ultimately, doctors are trained to meet the demands of patients and to improve patient care according to the Government's Health of the Nation targets.

Undergraduate medical education reflects many current changes in the NHS which impact on the resources available and changes in requirements from external stakeholders, such as the GMC, HEFCE and Health Authorities, which often make conflicting demands on organizations. In addition, the restructuring of health care in London has had a significant impact on the London medical schools, with all schools except one affected by mergers in the last five years as a response to the Tomlinson Report. ICSM is responding by maximizing on its own competencies, which include high research ratings, financial strength and stability and geographical location.

The partners and stakeholders

Imperial College School of Medicine: background and context

There are, at the time of writing, 26 undergraduate Medical Schools in the UK, which educate and train over 4000 doctors per year. Each of the medical schools is linked to a large teaching hospital and a number of associated district general hospitals and GP practices. Imperial College School of Medicine (ICSM) currently comprises the undergraduate St Mary's Hospital Medical School (SMHMS) and postgraduate National Heart and Lung Institute (NHLI). In late 1997, the undergraduate Charing Cross and Westminster Medical School (CXWMS) and Royal Postgraduate Medical School (RPMS) are due to merge with ICSM, as a result of negotiations with funding and health agencies. Funding was therefore secured for the building of a state-of-the-art Biomedical Sciences (BMS) block at South Kensington. The BMS building will be the focus for undergraduate teaching, linking all main sites by fibre-optic cable to enable distance learning and video-conferencing and using an extensive IT-based system for learning support. The new building will also house research staff from the existing Biology Department at Imperial College.

ICSM will also utilize three main hospital sites (Charing Cross, St

Mary's and Chelsea & Westminster) for clinical teaching. Students are also placed in a number of associated hospitals and general practices as part of their clinical experience. The new course has been designed along radical lines, and is the only mandatory six-year medical course in the UK outside Oxford and Cambridge, awarding all students an MBBS and BSc degree.

From October 1998, there will be a common curriculum with one ICSM cohort of 286 students studying across all sites. Historically, each of the four separate schools has had a Dean, a School Secretary and an autonomous management and administrative structure. The ICSM senior management team has been appointed and the new management structure will be flatter and information-based, this being a common response to organizational change. The Committee structure through which policy is established is in place.

UK medical schools have a stable market in terms of undergraduate students. Their main objective is to remain financially viable through the delivery of high quality education and training and by generating research income. The additional main strategic objectives of the new medical school are to bring the merger process into reality by 1997 and to introduce a new course in line with GMC recommendations, which also meets HEFCE requirements, into the new building by October 1998.

Internal stakeholders

There is stakeholder conflict over the above objectives. Although all staff recognize that the School has to remain financially stable, the ethos of academic autonomy means that there is, at present, little contractual control over staff workload. For example, basic medical science staff do not have contracts which stipulate their teaching load, which is currently managed at Departmental level. No central mechanism exists for identifying staff teaching, research or administrative load. There is a continuing tension between the demands of research and teaching (as in all HE institutions), which means that though the Medical School's main function is ostensibly to teach and train doctors, the drive to improve and maintain high research ratings is often a major force behind many management decisions. There are conflicts between the different partners in the merger process as individuals and groups come from very different backgrounds and academic disciplines, and there are strong site and institutional loyalties.

External stakeholders

The needs of external stakeholders have become increasingly impor- tant in altering the competitive environment. HE establishments, particularly the 'old' universities, perceive research as being of primary importance in terms of generating income through research grants, of raising the status of universities and of receiving more funding from HEFCE through the Research Assessment Exercise (RAE). This has promoted a culture of extreme competitiveness between HE institutions and their component departments, in that the RAE is a public document and establishments such as Oxford, Cambridge and Imperial College have tended to head the league tables. There is, therefore, extreme pressure on departments and individual staff to achieve grade 5 and 5* research ratings.

(a) The Higher Education Funding Council
UK medical schools have a quota of students allocated by HEFCE, based on employers' stated requirements and the estimated need for doctors at all grades over the next 20 years. Funding is based on the number of full-time equivalent students (FTEs) and Schools also receive tuition fees paid by LEAs for each student. HEFCE also provides funding for research allocated on the basis of the RAE, and Higher Education establishments with high ratings receive more than those with lower ones. The 'outputs' of ICSM therefore include the pro- duction of highly qualified manpower and research which serve as inputs to the productive sector of the economy. The 1987 White Paper on education specifies a third objective for HE – 'other social benefits'; these are often very difficult to quantify, particularly in a system in which traditionally hard work and fact transfer are highly emphasized.

HEFCE requires regular and reliable assessment of education to ensure accountability for the effective and responsible use of public funds; to inform institutions of the quality of the provision they offer; to facilitate the quality enhancement process and to provide information for others, including prospective students and employers. This feedback control loop requires HE institutions to measure per- formance by processing performance indicators (PIs) into useful information. HEFCE and other external stakeholders do not define the PIs (or evidence) but indicate the information they require from institutions.

There are often difficulties in defining PIs and, as Asch (1990) notes, this can be a barrier to strategic control. ICSM can easily define financial and quasi-financial measures, but 'softer' measures such as student satisfaction, and quality of the learning experience have not to date been rigorously defined by either undergraduate school.

The Committee of Vice Chancellors and Principals and University Grants Committee indicator sets for research selectivity comprise 39 indicators. These include staff and students numbers, income from research, and bibliometric measures, and form the basis of comparative indicators. Most of these are concerned with expenditure, and fail to relate to the relevant inputs or to measure 'value-added'. All HE institutions are regularly audited by various agencies and there are currently changes in the structure of the bodies which have monitored educational quality to date in that HEFCE and the Higher Education Quality Council are being subsumed under a single Quality Agency during 1997. The exact nature of the responsibilities of the new agency are not clear at the time of writing.

(b) The General Medical Council
Medical schools are also monitored by the GMC, which has a statutory obligation to ensure doctors are trained to appropriate standards and can, in extreme cases, revoke a school's licence to train doctors. In 1993, the GMC published *Tomorrow's Doctors*, which made specific recommendations for radical changes in undergraduate medical education. These were reinforced by a series of 'informal' visits to all Schools which aimed to measure how far they had implemented the recommendations. The five-year implementation period was supported by the Chief Medical Officer, Kenneth Calman, allocating funding to each School for facilitating this curricular change. The DoH also monitors the implementation of the recommendations through submission of four-monthly reports from each School.

The GMC recommended that basic medical sciences should not be learned separately from clinical training, as in traditional courses, but integrated, so that learning is centred around clinical conditions and situations. This has resource implications both in human and physical terms, as the resources used to deliver the existing courses are inap-propriate for the new curricula. There will be a multi-disciplinary approach to learning, with courses structured around body systems (e.g. cardiovascular) not around subject disciplines (e.g. biochemistry). This has immense implications for the traditional basic medical science departments, as they are discipline-based and currently 'own' their teaching. The new curriculum will also require departments to service specific course components by the provision of staff, rooms and equipment.

The GMC also moves towards a softer output model than earlier models, aiming to produce 'holders of concepts and principles that are transferable to a wide range of appropriate situations'. Interestingly, the GMC's proposed model, though inherently educational and delivered by universities, is very similar to categories of learning outcomes defined in a wide range of areas concerned with vocational training – intellectual skills; cognitive strategies; verbal information and motor skills and attitudes.

The GMC has shied away from defining national competencies or a national curriculum and clearly is unwilling to move towards national assessment standards as have the professional bodies of other countries, e.g. USA, Canada, Australia.

(c) The National Health Service Executive Regional Offices
In addition to HEFCE funding, money is allocated from the regional health authorities to NHS trusts and other providers in recognition of the excess costs to service departments for the clinical training of medical students. This funding is the Service Increment for Teaching (SIFT) and comprises an element for clinical placement of students. The SIFT allocation provides clinical directorates with a substantial amount of money. The directorates have come to regard this as a right, and nationally there was little accountability for this funding.

In the past few years, however, there has been a shift towards increasing transparency of the SIFT funding process and this has resulted in the introduction of rigorous monitoring of the quality of clinical teaching. The 1994 NHSE report *SIFT into the Future* recommended increased transparency of the process, and greater accountability in that medical schools were required formally to monitor and evaluate the allocation of SIFT on a departmental basis and submit annual reports to their NHSE Regional offices.

Funding has been allocated to schools for SIFT monitoring in terms of quantity and quality of clinical teaching, with the main aim of ensuring that schools and Health Authorities are getting value for money from service departments. This has led to the formulation of contracts between the NHSE and Trusts, co-signed by medical schools.

As the new structures are implemented, relationships change and tensions arise between the centre and operating divisions.

IT-based performance measures, for example, which will be introduced throughout ICSM, have caused resentment amongst NHS clinicians in the piloting of SIFT monitoring. This has been seen as changing the 'rules of the game', but it enables managers to retain and increase strategic control. The problems are compounded in monitoring teaching quality, as doctors have not been trained to teach, there is limited funding to carry out training, and staff turnover, particularly at below Consultant grade (i.e. Registrars) is very high. Some of these difficulties should be resolved through the implementation of the Calman recommendations on general specialist training, which aim to ensure that all doctors are given structured training and study leave throughout their specialist training period. These changes do, however, depend on the opportunity and willingness of career grade doctors to train undergraduates.

An additional difficulty is that although *SIFT into the Future* recommended a 'steady state' of funding allocation for the next five years, the GMC recommends that Schools aim to base at least 20% and ideally up to 40% of clinical teaching in the community and General Practice to reflect the reality of UK health care.

Currently, ICSM has less than 5% of clinical placement time allocated to community teaching, and a large shift within three years from hospital-based clinical teaching to community could have a huge impact on some clinical departments. This has to be managed centrally so as to avoid major difficulties for departments.

Project planning methodology

The process of strategy formation

Overall strategy is formulated by the Rector of Imperial College and the Imperial senior management team. Undergraduate Medical Curriculum strategy is steered by two senior committees. One (the Medical Curriculum Executive Group, MCEG) comprises senior representatives from all five participating institutions who have responsibility for medical education, clinical or basic science. The MCEG formulates policy and makes decisions on resource allocation. The other group is the Joint Education Committee (JEC). The JEC acts as a forum for discussion and debate on the detail of course design and implementation and makes recommendations to the MCEG.

The strategic development of ICSM is managed as part of the overall Imperial College strategy. It is incremental, and policy-making is adaptive as the structure has to fit the needs of the new course, and vice versa.

Formulation and implementation are inter-related (Quinn, 1989) and it is often the internal processes such as employee capabilities, co-ordination and leadership which are bottlenecks to implementation, as described below. The organizational development has been partly emergent, for example, the divisions and departmental structures and staffing are not yet finalised as this relates partly to curriculum design and partly to research commitments.

Project planning

The Medical Education Unit (MEU) was established in 1993 and is the executive unit of the committees concerned with undergraduate medical education. It produces course documentation and co-ordinates the detailed curriculum development process, and in particular it co-ordinates a vast amount of information. Information is seen as both a resource and intelligence. Our policy is to be open with information and ensure that those in need of specific information receive it, whilst others are not deluged. The staff of the MEU are essentially the project management team on a day-to-day basis, though they obviously report to senior staff and through the Committee structures. The MEU has used an organizational development approach and specific project management techniques in developing curriculum strategy, using team building and external facilitators as change agents. ICSM can be seen as organic; its capability is in the process of being developed, and political and status systems are changing as staff loyalties and goals are threatened.

Kotter and Schlesinger (1979) suggest involving people in change to ensure ownership. At present, staff are not always consulted or involved in the overall changes and this leads to resentment and potential problems for implementing strategies. The curriculum development project can be seen as having major areas, some of which are directly related to developing a new curriculum (development of course materials, for example) and others which are essential for the effective implementation of the new course, such as the development of an IT-based management information system, staff training and development and a system of academic counselling and guidance and pastoral care for students.

Originally there were two Units, one on the CXWMS site and one on the St Mary's site. It was unclear at that stage whether the two Medical Schools would be merging but it was decided at senior level that, as both Schools had to consider the implementation of the recommendations in *Tomorrow's Doctors* on their curricula, the process of curriculum development should be carried out as a joint project. Funding was obtained from within each School to establish the facilities and a day-to-day budget.

This was considerably enhanced by the Department of Health providing funding to all UK Medical Schools (and later to Dental Schools) to facilitate curriculum change. The decision by the DoH to support the GMC recommendations in this way was instrumental in the radical changes which have been made to undergraduate medical education since 1993. The funding was made to Schools specifically for the appointment of curriculum facilitators, appointed either from within the current staffing of a School or externally.

The contribution to the curriculum development projects of the curriculum facilitators cannot be underestimated. The facilitators established a national network which still exists for support and guidance, and which acts as a forum for the exchange of ideas and expertise. Many of the facilitators could be viewed as 'credible outsiders', bringing educational input into a process which traditionally has had a course clearly divided into pre-clinical basic medical sciences taught by academics and a clinical training period following an apprenticeship model. An external facilitator was appointed at CXWMS and the existing MEU Administrator at St Mary's was appointed as their curriculum facilitator. The planning process was overseen by the Joint Education Committee until the formation of the Medical Curriculum Executive Group in 1996. The JEC determined the overall structure of the new course in late 1993 and allocated time to each of the three main elements of the MBBS course.

Curriculum development is an iterative process. There are many 'problem owners' and stakeholders who all need to be consulted at the appropriate stage. The project can be seen as having the three stages of a Systems Intervention Strategy – Planning, Design and Implementation – with clear loops back to key stakeholders to facilitate the process. In the planning stage, the MEU staff from both Schools worked together on the details of the process under the Directorship of a nominated academic from St Mary's.

Great care was taken at this stage to ensure that both Schools were represented equally on all committees and working groups. This was very effective in ensuring ownership of the new course and also that staff from both Schools could start to meet and work together on joint tasks. This was instrumental in beginning to break down some of the barriers between the Schools. Staff of the MEU met regularly and produced discussion documents for the JEC concerning core content, course philosophies and proposals for development strategy. Each of the main areas of the course – Systems and Topics, Doctor and Patient, Clinical Experience and the BSc – were co-ordinated by either one or two MEU members who were accountable for the progress of that specific area. A course design team was established for each of the main areas with a remit to develop it, and each team had two convenors drawn from each School. The sixteen Systems and Topics courses had individual course design teams, as it was determined that this was the area which should spearhead the development process.

As the course was to be integrated both horizontally (in that basic medical sciences and clinical science were to be taught together in a multi-disciplinary approach) and vertically (in that clinical experience was to be available from the first year and basic medical sciences to continue throughout the course), all design teams were representative of clinical specialities and academic disciplines. The emphasis placed on this strategy reflected the OD approach, using methods such as team working, focus groups, consultative exercises and widespread surveys, involvement of key players, including staff at all levels and student representatives, and establishing effective communication links. Instructions were written by the MEU to course convenors concerning various aspects of course development and planning; this was to ensure a standardized process and to guide the teams on how to proceed with their work. It was decided that the course would be 'objective-led'; many teachers had never been involved in course planning and it was felt that, despite the potential rigidity of this approach, it was essential that clear learning outcomes were defined from the outset. The curriculum facilitators attended each meeting to actively support the teams and give direct help and training if necessary.

Many convenors and team members required training sessions on specific topics such as objective writing and problem-based learning, and these were delivered by the MEU in response to their requests. The MEU has now appointed a staff member with the remit of staff training and development as it is felt that this is essential to support the process.

The curriculum development process was quite simple (if not easy) in the early stages and the project was moving forward within the planned timescale. In late 1995, it became clear that the proposed merger was actually going to take place and by 1997, the new Imperial College School of Medicine would comprise two under-graduate and two postgraduate Schools under one umbrella. This decision had immense impact on the curriculum project in that many of the structures and processes 'froze' whilst the new Principal was appointed, whilst the management structure of the School was being planned and whilst staff were absorbing the impact on their work.

In addition to this, many staff were to move to the new BMS building at South Kensington from their hospital sites and the proposed structure and staffing profile of the School is not yet clear at the time of writing. The curriculum project thus went through a stage of theoretical activity in that participants were very engrossed in the theory of education and learning and aimed to design courses around ideal practice. This was not all negative, as the project team used this period to train and educate staff on these issues, many aspects of which were new to them. This indicates that a project management team must be prepared to be responsive to people and be prepared to modify and be flexible on the sequencing of different phases of the project. In a very complex project, some aspects are not achieved sequentially, but in parallel and so long as the project is plotted using methods like critical path analysis to identify the key activities (using IT-based project management systems, if appropriate), there should be flexibility in achieving outcomes within the overall plan.

The project then moved into a stage of limbo in which much resentment was encountered and many staff, even those who were formerly most enthusiastic, became very reluctant to participate as there was so much uncertainty due to the merger. The MEU took time out from the detailed planning and actively stood down course design teams whilst it overviewed the whole course in the light of the development process to date, and the proposed ICSM structure.

This stage also saw the establishment of the MCEG and much more involvement from Imperial College staff and staff from the post-graduate institutions who had not been involved in undergraduate teaching or course development until then. It was decided that the MEU should be relocated and restructured as a combined unit on the main Imperial College South Kensington campus.

This gave a clear message to all staff that the future of under-graduate medical education was being led by Imperial College School of Medicine, and not by one or other undergraduate School. Once the revised overview of the course had been through the various com-mittees, the course teams were revived and in some cases re-con-figured. They were given a new task with a very clear time-frame – to complete their course planning so that detailed proposals were available in order that the MEU could define and allocate human and physical resources. The project, which originally was defined with a clear mission (to develop a new course in line with the GMC recom-mendations) then moved into a very complex stage in which boundaries and lines of communication and accountability became very blurred. There were innumerable occasions in which the cur-riculum process was halted or constrained whilst individuals were appointed, or whilst structures or procedural mechanisms were established in the new School.

MacMillan (1985) notes the nature of political strategy formulation, identifying allies and opponents, lobbying, negotiating, developing informal relationships and a network of contacts.

ICSM's strategy, and that of the MEU, utilizes all of these mech-anisms as it is a highly political environment.

In some ways, the project can be seen as acting as a vehicle for change and the curriculum development process can be used to drive through some of the broader changes deemed necessary for the suc-cess of the new School. The course is designed to reflect the strengths of Imperial College and in particular the new School of Medicine.

The main impact on the specific project was slippage in the planned delivery of the new course; it was originally intended to deliver a joint course in 1996, but this was changed to October 1998. A major diffi-culty for the project team in the MEU was that they were continually being drawn into developing areas which were not directly related to the curriculum. These included the teaching facilities in the new BMS building, advising on the IT infrastructure, resource planning and management and the Management Information Systems required for the new School.

The core project team was expanded with the appointment of additional full-time staff, as it was quickly recognized that full-time academic staff and clinicians did not have either the time or the specific expertise to carry out many of the activities needed. This highlights the need for continual monitoring of a project and the need for modifications wherever necessary. Many of the UK medical schools have encountered slippage in the planning, design and implementation of their new curricula; the process is very complicated, involving many people who must have ownership of the new course, supported by a staff training and development programme to facilitate the introduction of new teaching/learning techniques. Introducing new medical courses in line with the GMC recommendations has proved very difficult even for medical schools with a relatively stable structure; to do so at a time of merger and whilst moving to a new site has proved immensely complex.

Implementation and monitoring

Implementation

The new course is planned for delivery in October 1998. The curriculum project itself is keeping to the planned time frame and the four elements of the course are, at the time of writing, being planned in detail. Because there are two undergraduate courses currently running successfully, the expertise to deliver a medical undergraduate course is available across the School.

Strategy should be contingent, responding to change with strategies that most fit the organization. Force field analysis reveals the tension between pull factors maintaining the status quo (geographic location of sites, staff attitudes, organizational paradigms and traditional staff teaching skills) and factors pushing for change: external stakeholders, competition with other medical schools and technological changes.

A contingency approach has led the project outcomes to be fairly flexible in that we know that a course will be delivered in 1998 which differs substantially from the current courses. It may be that the new course is not completely ready in 1998, but courses are always subject to review and change and an incremental approach is appropriate here. It is essential to consider a planned series of outcomes within a fluid timeframe.

In some cases, action may be brought forward, for example, some course teams have taken the decision to introduce their new courses two years ahead of the new MBBS BSc course, in order to pilot content and methods of teaching and learning. In other cases, action may be delayed, usually reflecting changes in the wider College environment or particular local difficulties.

The rationale behind this approach is based on the immense changes which are taking place for staff from 1997 to 1999. The present basic science departments are to be merged and re-organized into divisions based on current research divisions, not subject disciplines. The clinical academic departments will also fit into this new divisional structure. The matrix management structure will overlay the site-based activities of the four institutions; these will always remain semi-autonomous, as their activities are closely linked to NHS service activities. Substantive and procedural rationality, though 'bounded', can be seen as operating in a systems model of the organization which stresses the dynamics of relations between the component parts and the organization and its environment. In many cases, the new Divisional structure will service the new System-based course more effectively than the current Departmental structure, but will essentially support academic research. The success of the course rests not only on the course materials, content and assessment structure but also on the willingness and ability of staff to deliver it. It may well be that the stress of changes in 1998, and the practicalities of relocating and restructuring of work practices has a much greater impact on staff morale than is currently anticipated.

The academic staff of the new school will be organized according to their research and their teaching; these will not be the same in most cases. Currently, there are immense problems with staff delivering good quality teaching. Research commitments take priority; if staff are labelled as 'academic', they are counted towards the RAE and this leads to good teachers being pulled away from teaching, and those with poor research records being given more teaching, whether appropriate or not. HEFCE's teaching quality assessments do not have the same financial 'teeth' as the RAE, and because of the changes in the undergraduate curriculum, medicine will not be assessed until 1998 onwards. The teaching quality assessment will be published, but the moves are towards self-assessment and continual review rather than rewarding or penalizing establishments financially. This tends to maintain the status of teaching as lower than that of research. There are, however, competing forces for change. Schools are therefore under increasing pressure to introduce not only radical new courses, but also new methods of teaching, learning and assessment. There is currently 'cultural lag', as structural change is delayed, and there is lag with the training and development of staff.

If the new course is to succeed, there is a need to standardize norms and skills and develop relevant promotional and incentive strategies. Mintzberg (1983) suggests that using liaison devices to encourage communication across specialist boundaries (avoiding 'groupthink') helps to create co-ordinated strategy. These changes cannot be made without altering the organizational structure and control systems. The curriculum development process has been very successful in providing a focus for liaison, but this must be developed and embedded into the formal organizational structure.

Monitoring

As described above, due to the collegiate management structure at Imperial College, the project is monitored through the MEU being responsible to senior staff and accountable through the Committee structures to Imperial College senior management. A conscious decision was made to involve key stakeholders from all participating institutions on a number of curriculum committees. The curriculum development process has been made as transparent as is possible within a highly politicized environment. The MEU, as the project team, has been given delegated powers to make day-to-day decisions and any areas which need further clarification or resolving are taken to the JEC and then to the MCEG if necessary. The project team monitors the activity of individuals and the process as a whole on a regular basis, meeting weekly as a minimum to ensure co-ordination of the process.

The two senior members of the MEU have responsibility for ensuring that the curriculum development process 'fits' with the overall strategy and policies of Imperial College. The day-to-day management of the project involves setting clear boundaries around activities of individuals and groups, ensuring that tasks are planned in a logical and co-ordinated way, that action plans are set and reviewed regularly with modifications made as appropriate. The project as a whole must have clear objectives and each activity must be clearly linked to the achievement of the overall objectives.

Conclusion and project outcomes

Apart from the 300 staff directly involved in planning the new course, staff are still site-based, with site loyalties and cultures. The BMS building will not be ready for occupancy until April 1998 and until then staff will not be in the new divisions. The new course commences in October 1998, which only gives six months for staff to move sites, set up research, form new working relationships and finalize preparation for the new course. In addition, some staff will work on split sites in 1998 as the existing courses may still be running at both SMHMS and CXWMS. The uncertainty over the changes is very threatening for staff at all levels, with the restructuring of the current departments into a new Divisional structure. It is essential that the organizational structure is clearly defined and communicated in the near future and that negotiations with staff affected are carried out sensitively. Power relationships between individuals and departments have the potential to sabotage the planned strategy in many ways, and care must be taken to avoid this.

ICSM is well-placed to achieve its aim of becoming one of the strongest medical schools in Europe. The curriculum is designed to meet the requirements of all internal and external stakeholders, it has in-built performance indicators, an excellent IT-based MIS and some of the highest-rated research departments in the country. It 'fits' with the environment and its strategic objectives have been clearly defined with reference to environmental change. The importance of training staff so that they are equipped with the new teaching, administrative and IT skills needed, should not be under-estimated; the present workforce does not have the skills to deliver the new course in its entirety.

Dissemination and consultation

There is regular dissemination on the progress of the curriculum development project. From the outset, there have been regular newsletters detailing plans and outlining the process which have been distributed to all recognized teachers and other key internal and external stakeholders. These newsletters have invited participation and acted as a focus for staff from all partner organizations to be involved with the new course. In addition to the medical education bulletins, Imperial College produces the fortnightly *Reporter* which informs staff on all aspects of life at Imperial College, including the new School of Medicine. The building projects at Imperial produce *Hard Hat*, which informs staff on progress on the new Biomedical Sciences building at South Kensington.

The Medical Education Unit team have given presentations concerning the new course to all Academic Departments at ICSM, again encouraging participation and inviting comments on the new course and input into its development and delivery. The aim is to involve people from all participating institutions who are interested in undergraduate medical education in the development process and in delivering the new course. Other key groups, such as NHS committees, have been targeted and all the clinical sites have been visited both formally and informally. The aim of this wide dissemination is to ensure that individuals and groups have been given the opportunity for involvement in the design of the new course. Prior to the appointment of the Principal of ICSM, Professor Christopher Edwards, an 'Awayday' was held for all staff directly involved in course development. This was very effective at updating people on the work of other groups and enabling co-ordinators of the discrete course elements to locate their course within the complete structure. Regular communication with staff is vital, ensuring that NHS staff on many different hospital sites remain in touch with the very rapid developments has been one of the most difficult challenges concerning communication.

Changes resulting from project outcomes

At the time of writing, there have been few changes made as a result of project outcomes as the project is not yet completed. Due to the iterative nature of the project management strategy, the curriculum development project has impacted on the merger project and vice versa. This highlights the need to fit the project management strategy into the overall organizational strategy, that is, the 'near' environment as well as the 'far'. Issues indirectly associated with the project have stimulated staff to implement changes in teaching practice, introducing new topics into the current courses, new teaching/learning methods and new assessment methods, for example, and the excitement generated by the curriculum changes have raised staff awareness of teaching and learning issues.

This has happened nationally as a result of the widespread involvement of medical schools in curriculum development and change management programmes. The curriculum development project can therefore be seen as both a discrete project in itself with clear outcomes and as providing a vehicle for wider changes in organizational structure and practice.

References

Asch, D. (1990) in *Performance Measurement and Evaluation*, Macmillan Educ., Basingstoke, 1995.

General Medical Council, *Tomorrow's Doctors*, 1993 HEQC Guidelines on Quality Assurance, 1996.

Kotter, J.P. and Schlesinger, L.A. (1979), in Asch, D. and Bowman, C. (eds) *Readings in Strategic Management*, Macmillan, Basingstoke, 1989.

MacMillan, I.C. (1985), Strategy Formulation: Political Concepts (St. Paul MN: West).

Mintzberg, H. (1983), in Asch, D. and Bowman, C. (eds) *Readings in Strategic Management*, Macmillan, Basingstoke, 1989.

Quinn, J.B. (1989), in Asch, D. and Bowman, C. (eds) *Readings in Strategic Management*, Macmillan, Basingstoke, 1989.

Case Study 2

The community hospitals development project

Brendan Mc Cormack, BSc (Hons) Nursing, DPSN, PGCEA, RNT, RGN, RMN
Programme Director (Community Hospitals, Nursing Homes & Gerontological Nursing), Royal College of Nursing Institute, Oxford & Oxfordshire Community Health NHS Trust

Background

Oxfordshire Community Health NHS Trust (OCHT) is one of seven health care Trusts in the County of Oxfordshire. It serves a population of 500 000 people with 'general' health care services (does not include mental health, obstetrics or learning disability services) including community nursing, therapy services, dental services and community hospitals. There are 12 community hospitals in Oxfordshire and 11 of these are part of the Oxfordshire Community Trust. We have community hospitals at Abingdon, Bicester, Burford, Chipping Norton, Didcot, Oxford City, Thame, Wallingford, Wantage, Watlington and Witney. The vision for the Community Hospitals of Oxfordshire is to create a local hospital structure that meets the health care needs of local populations and is responsive to, enhances and compliments the work of Primary Health Care teams.

This project focused on the development of the services provided by community hospitals and the identification of ways that community hospitals could expand their services, in order to turn the vision of 'local hospitals' into a reality. The project took place over one year. The drive for such changes arose from the Community Trust and the

Oxfordshire Health Authority, who had both published their proposals for such developments. These proposals provided the major focus of the project.

In addition, reviews of Community Hospitals undertaken by both the Trust and Oxfordshire Health Authority demonstrated a commitment to the service from GPs and their desire for the quality of care delivered to be improved. Development work being undertaken by the Community Hospitals of Oxfordshire, particularly the work of the Community Hospitals Nursing Development Unit provided an appropriate foundation on which to build. The Community Hospitals Nursing Development Unit (CHNDU) had been in existence for four years. During that time, its focus had been on developing clinical nursing practice within a corporate framework throughout the 11 hospitals. This framework was being developed to incorporate multidisciplinary working and the development of rehabilitation services. As a part of the development framework and to ensure that developments related to actual practice, the CHNDU devised an audit programme to establish a baseline of the quality of care from which focused development work could be implemented. While the audit programme was nursing focused, it was not nursing specific, as it encapsulated issues about the context of care and relationships with other members of the multidisciplinary team. The audit programme was based on principles of:

- staff ownership of the process and outcomes of audit;
- facilitation of changes through the use of adult education approaches leading to changes being secured in practice.

While all of these developments had helped focus the need for the organizational development of the community hospitals, four key drivers for change were identified that reflected both changes in policy and future plans for the provision of health care:

1. An increased investment in the infrastructure of community hospitals in order for them to achieve their maximum potential;
2. Opportunities available to maximize capacity;
3. Oxfordshire Health Authority's Stroke Strategy;
4. Community Care changes.

Overall, the central aim of the project was to maximize the productivity of community hospitals, develop their vital contribution to the range of health care options available and ensure that they remained a viable option as a part of health care provision in localities.

Terms of reference

The terms of reference for the project were determined by the drivers for change as previously indicated. The project had a six-month time scale and therefore a realistic project plan needed to be devised so that priority areas could be achieved. Therefore, the expected outcome of the project was:

Through undertaking key developments, create a cultural shift from 11 individual community hospitals to a 'local hospital' structure with 350 in-patient beds and a range of out-patient services that meet the health care needs of local populations.

The identified key objectives were:

1. To examine and develop methods of improving equity of access;
2. To improve productivity of all aspects of hospital provision;
3. To have common standards, protocols and monitoring and reporting structures across the 11 sites;
4. To propose the optimum mix of nursing, paramedical and medical practice and approaches to achieving this;
5. To create more formal links with other agencies.

Methodology

A critical pathway approach was taken. Each area of work had a project plan with key milestones identified as appropriate to the project design. The project drew extensively on existing work where appropriate. For example, many hospitals had admission criteria available. These were analysed, and appropriate criteria identified and used in the formation of protocols. People were consulted widely throughout the project. Processes of consultation used included:

- Consensus workshop with key staff from OCHT, Oxford Radcliffe Hospitals (ORH) Trust, Oxfordshire Health, Social Services, General Practitioners and Community Health Council. In order to validate the protocols and standards developed, 'experts' from the above services were selected to attend an all day workshop. Draft standards and protocols were reviewed, critiqued and validated.

- Focused group interview with clinical leaders. F and G grade nurses who fulfilled the role of 'Development Facilitator' for the Community Hospitals Development Unit were selected for interview. A further representative sample of Physiotherapists and Occupational Therapists employed in the hospitals were chosen. Two focused groups were formed. Interviews were conducted by the Project Manager, a Hospital Manager, the Trust's Head of Physiotherapy and a GP. A structured interview schedule was used.
- Focused group interviews with General Practitioners. A 10% stratified random sample of all GPs with admitting rights to community hospitals was selected. Stratification criteria included, practice population size, distance of the practice from the hospital and fundholding/non-fundholding. Three groups were formed, representing different geographical areas of the Trust. Interviews were conducted jointly by the project manager and a GP. A total of 28 GPs were interviewed using a semi-structured interview schedule.
- Questionnaire to members of the Local Medical Committee (LMC) prior to attendance at the meeting.
- Individual discussions with specialist medical consultants.
- Presentation of project work to project board for refinement, critique and validation.

Outcomes

The original intentions of the project were realized as intended. Demonstrable improvements in the level of collaboration both within the Community Trust and across Trusts was evident as a result of this work. While this was clearly evident, it was difficult to quantify this and its impact on care. Much enthusiasm and commitment to co-operation between Trusts to secure the implementation of the project outcomes was achieved. Similar levels of co-operation were evident through emerging work with Oxfordshire Social Services. The changes in practice and service delivery achieved through this project, resulted in a commitment by Oxfordshire Health Authority to increase its investment in community hospital services. This investment helped to secure changes that occurred in the organization and delivery of services in the Community Hospitals. The central aim of these changes was to increase productivity and effectiveness of the services delivered. The outcomes derived from the project focus on three areas:

- Equity of productivity and provision;
- Commonality of procedures, development of protocols;
- Clinical practice: issues and proposals.

1. Equity of productivity and provision

Of crucial importance was the creation of staffing and organizational structures in each hospital that were based on equitable levels of resourcing, so that services were not delivered according to historical resources, but instead were based on established and agreed criteria. Previous reviews of community hospitals identified that there were areas of inequity in resourcing between hospitals.

Using the criteria of hospital activity and average dependency levels, a skill mix ratio has been established for each hospital. The results of this work have been used to inform the allocation of new investment. Those areas with appropriate skill mix, identified population need based on current demands and capacity for expansion were highlighted and thus targeted for increased activity. This work has further been used to identify productivity targets for the service.

From an analysis of current activity per bed in all hospitals, it was possible to identify the relative productivity of each hospital. From this data, the activity gain needed in each hospital to create equitable levels of productivity across sites was identified. The activity per bed of each hospital was compared against the actual populations served. From this data comparisons could be drawn between the productivity of the hospital relative to the population served. By taking the average range of activity, and identifying the areas of least and most activity, it was possible to identify a range that would lead to equitable levels of productivity based on the contract currency.

2. Commonality of procedures: development of protocols

The focus of this work was the development of agreed organizational and clinical protocols for:

- admission and refusal of admission;
- transfer of care from acute sector;

- discharge planning;
- respite care provision;
- continence;
- verbal prescribing of medicines;
- resuscitation.

A review of available admission policies demonstrated differences in approaches to the acceptance of admissions and criteria for acceptance. While most hospitals were using an admissions policy that had been developed in 1984, it was being interpreted in various ways by the hospitals. There were further differences in prioritizing between direct admissions from home and those transferred from secondary care. Evidence existed from both secondary care and community hospital staff of a lack of understanding of each other's work. The development of common protocols agreed between all hospitals was seen as a way of addressing some of these problems. Following consultation, as described in the methodology, protocols for admission and refusal of admission, transfer of care from secondary care, discharge planning and respite care provision have been established. The formation and implementation of these protocols offers the community hospitals and other providers, consistency in approaches to practice. They include directions for development (*e.g. patient-held multi-disciplinary records* and *pre-admission assessment of patients' respite care needs*). They further focus on collaboration between Trusts and Social Services and provide opportunities for audit and research.

A number of implementation actions were agreed and are in operation:

- A referral form was devised for use by community hospital staff in discussing referrals with the Acute Trusts and for guiding decisions in accepting admissions.
- Guidelines were devised for staff in the Acute Trusts, to help them make decisions about appropriate transfers to community hospitals and the information required for successful transfer.
- Education sessions for community hospital and acute hospital staff.
- Development of the Community Liaison Service to:
  Jointly working with Oxfordshire Social Services and Oxfordshire Health Authority in the ongoing monitoring of service delivery and its impact on social care provision.

The protocols were audited as follows:

- quarterly review of referral forms;
- auditing of assessments and transfers by the liaison service.
- annual audit of respite care provision, including:
  - number of clients;
  - reason for provision of respite care;
- retrospective documentation audit;
- Monitoring of delayed discharges through the minimum data set procedures.

3. Clinical practice: Issues and proposals

In order to establish if there were links between the levels of productivity and the quality of care, the data derived from an audit of clinical practice in Community Hospitals was analysed.

To develop the audit tool, an extensive review of the literature was undertaken, from which valid and reliable instruments (where available) were chosen. From this, 11 audit themes were identified and an audit package devised. A development facilitator in each hospital who was trained in the use of the audit package and facilitation skills was identified to act as the internal auditor. The development facilitator was also responsible for the organization, collection and dissemination of data and the formation of the ongoing development action plan.

Each clinical area had the audit undertaken over a one-week period. The audit was conducted jointly by the internal auditor and an external auditor from within the Trust.

Results

Analysis of the audit data demonstrated that the quality of care as determined by the audit did not have a direct relationship with productivity. It did not follow that those hospitals with low admission rates and high turnover intervals had better quality overall. The issue appeared to be more concerned with the availability of a multidisciplinary team, the way members of the multidisciplinary team worked together and the need for an approach to care based on multidisciplinary rehabilitation. This resulted in the development of an interdisciplinary rehabilitation strategy.

Investing in service development

The recognition of the need for key stakeholders (purchasers and providers) to agree on the model of community hospital to be provided and to continue to develop methods of collaborative working to achieve this was an important outcome from this project. While all those who participated in the project had their ideas about what the community hospital of the future would look like, there was an identified need for this view to be further refined and agreed. The work on the development of protocols had begun a process of collaboration that proved worthwhile in terms of achieving outcomes from patient care and ensuring that appropriate patient care is delivered in the most appropriate place. An inter-Trust working group was established as a result of this work and this acted as an example of how collaboration and co-operation could break down barriers and generate structures and processes to enhance the movement of patients through the health care system.

Community hospitals themselves are committed to becoming more effective and productive in their work. The work that was undertaken in creating equitable resourcing and the audit of clinical practice with resulting practice changes demonstrated this commitment. Since the project began, changes in occupancy figures have begun to be identified and a greater understanding of the need to balance patient dependency with productivity has been achieved. The new resources committed by Oxfordshire Health Authority have further enhanced this work by the development of rehabilitation services. The recognition of much of this work in the service specification developed by Oxfordshire Health Authority further recognizes a commitment to collaboration towards the delivery of an effective service.

Summary

The work begun during this project and the outcomes achieved have been developed into a programme of clinical practice and organizational development. This programme is a collaboration between the Trust and the Royal College of Nursing Institute. An ethos of development has been established, that recognizes clinical practice and organizational development as central to the delivery of a quality service.

This work informs and is informed by strategic developments, in particular:

- The Development of Intermediate Care Services;
- Oxfordshire Health Authority's Stroke Strategy;
- Oxfordshire Health Authority's Disability Strategy;
- The Primary-Secondary Interface.

Our community hospitals are at the forefront of these developments, which focus on locality-based services working in partnership with specialist providers.

This project provided an opportunity to consolidate some aspects of work and develop a framework for the strategic development of community hospital services. As such it 'never ends' but continues to respond to and influence changing health and social care demands.

Case study 3

The district nurse development project

Janet Allen, RNMH, BA (Hons), Hull and Holderness Community
Health NHS Trust

Background

During 1995, four research projects were undertaken across our
Community Trusts. The projects were:

- a health needs analysis;
- implementation of a joint documentation care file (a file on
  individual patients, shared by both health and social services);
- investigation into District Nurse working;
- investigation into the needs of an out of hours service.

Each of these had recommendations for practice, and a meeting took
place between the Director of Nursing, Research and Development Co-
ordinator and the Professional Head for District Nursing to agree on a
way forward for the systematic implementation of the recommendations. From this meeting, an outline proposal was written for a six-
month project to progress the recommendations into a model for
District Nursing, and for this model to be piloted across teams within
the Trust.

Setting up the project

The key stakeholders were identified by identifying who would be most
affected by the project, who would be in a position to 'escalate' or

manage problems, who would need to manage the project and be its sponsor in terms of finance and commitment. Membership and roles were as follows:

- Director of Nursing (project sponsor, and in a position to escalate solutions);
- Professional Head for District Nursing (planning, implementation and escalation);
- Research and Development Co-ordinator (project manager);
- Social Services Manager (stakeholder in care-file, and escalation for social service staff);
- Senior Lecturer in District Nursing (academic advice);
- Clinical Team Managers of District Nursing Teams (implementation of project objectives through the teams).

In addition, the Steering Group's role was to communicate and disseminate the progress of the project, and anticipate and report problems to the project manager who would ensure the schedule was adhered to or adapted pro-actively where possible.

Recruitment of teams to the project was an important phase, and this was done through a workshop involving all the District Nursing Managers where the purpose, aims of the project and resources needed by teams were revealed. At the end of the workshop, five managers and teams volunteered to take part, and the structure of the project was in place. As the project would mean extra work within already stretched teams, it was crucial that the teams showed initial enthusiasm and commitment by volunteering.

The Project Team consisted of the project manager, two part-time project officers, and a part-time research administrator.

The Steering Group met monthly and the Project team weekly.

Implementation

The model devised for the teams consisted of a health needs analysis being undertaken simultaneously with a profile of the District Nursing teams, and the implementation of the Joint Care File. These activities constituted the first stage of the project. The second stage involved combining information from the health needs analysis and the District Nurse profile, with needs and strengths being identified as a result.

The third stage was identifying areas for further investigation and development of practice.

The final stage was an evaluation of the project and each team.

Each District Nursing team had a link person from the Project Team to assist them through each stage.

A Project Team workshop was organized to define the scope of the project, produce a risk analysis, define objectives, tasks and activities, identify resources needed, establish responsibilities and accountability, and draw up a schedule.

In addition to the overall project schedule, a timetable and activity chart was drawn up for each element of the model, for each team. This sounds complex, but actually served to clarify timing and activities, and each team member was aware at all stages of the progress made and achievement of objectives.

At the Steering Group meetings, the overall project schedule was reviewed, with progress against objectives being one of the main agenda items. At the weekly Project Team meeting, each activity chart for the teams and model was reviewed, problems were identified and either solved or referred to the Steering Group.

Progress

At an interim review, 60% of the objectives and activities were found to be on schedule or had already been achieved. It might be interesting at this point to identify some of the problems which arose.

(a) The link person for one of the teams had to be changed halfway through the project because of an inappropriate match between the culture of the team and the interpersonal skills of the project officer.

(b) A heavy rate of sickness in one of the District Nursing teams resulted in them being one month behind on the project schedule.

(c) Another District Nursing team changed managers, and it was negotiated that they started on the project a month later than everyone else.

(d) The social services representative attended one Steering Group meeting only, and stayed at arm's length throughout the project, seriously affecting the implementation of the Joint Care File. Despite escalation, this problem was not successfully resolved.

(e) 200 questionnaires from one team from the health needs analysis were misplaced for a month.

Outcomes

The aims of the project were achieved, after a re-negotiation of deadlines extended the project by one month, with additional resources allocated. District Nurse teams throughout the Trust are now implementing the model on which to build their service delivery and planning, and further work is being undertaken with social services to implement the Joint Care File.

Dissemination of the project was via bulletins to District Nurses, presentations to Senior Management Board meetings and District Nursing teams. Ongoing support to District Nursing teams is being negotiated in terms of analysis of questionnaires.

The outcomes of the project are being integrated into a strategy for District Nursing and being fed into the objective-setting process for each team.

Case Study 4

Digital Media in Nurse Education (DiNET) – vocational language skills for healthcare workers

Ray Kirtley, European Awareness Project, Humberside Local Education Authority

The origins of the project

The planning process for the project took place in the early part of 1995. It was at this time that Carol Ludvigsen was appointed by the Hull and Holderness Health Trust as European Co-ordinator. Part of her role was to meet others in the area who were performing a similar function but in other sectors. This took her to both of the local universities, Hull and Humberside, to the Training and Enterprise Council and to the local education authority.

Humberside Local Education Authority had taken the farsighted step of appointing a European Awareness Co-ordinator in 1990 and by 1995 the postholder, Ray Kirtley, had gained wide experience of European projects. Several of these projects had a technical dimension and by 1995 the European Awareness initiative was virtually integrated into Humberside TVEI. The Technical and Vocational Education Initiative, now ended in most parts of the country, was funded through local education authorities by the Government Office. It enabled LEAs to pilot curriculum-led initiatives mostly involving the application of science and technology. In Humberside the TVEI team had been pioneers in producing CD-ROMS and associated resources for use in schools by using the expertise of practising teachers in the authoring process. Some of the existing titles demonstrated the use of CD-ROM technology for language learning.

It was this combination of personnel, experience and circumstances which led to the idea for the project. The need for the project was already clear to Ray Kirtley from his background work on career patterns and worker mobility in the European Union. Carol Ludvigsen confirmed that workers in the healthcare sector were especially immobile due to a lack of vocational language skills. She also knew of few products or schemes which set out to address this deficiency.

Therefore it was this combination of expertise in the health and education sectors coupled with a supportive and informed technical environment which led to the conception of the project. Both of the main actors were aware of the new Leonardo programme and were able to construct the project within its parameters.

Who were the partners and stakeholders and how were they identified?

The identification of the partners was a joint exercise which relied on contacts known to Carol Ludvigsen and, to a lesser extent, Ray Kirtley. Several factors were taken into account but the key to the choice was diversity. Both potential co-ordinators took the view that the project would be best served if the partners came from a combination of nurse education and linguistic training backgrounds. All the partners who were approached agreed to take part in the project giving a final structure as follows:

Strategic Co-ordinator	Project Co-ordinator	Project Worker
Ray Kirtley European Awareness Project Humberside LEA	Carol Ludvigsen Hull & Holderness Community Health Trust	Kim Dent Brown Hull & Holderness Community Health Trust
Technical Director	**Audio Visual**	**Audio Visual**
Ian Dolphin Curriculum Development Humberside LEA	Richard Garbutt Curriculum Development Humberside LEA	Mary Rogers Media Studies Department Grimsby College

Co-partner — Spain	Co-partner — Spain	Partner — Germany
Ramón Camaño-Puig Escola Universitaria d'Infermeria Universitat de Valencia	Jordi Piqué Escola Universitaria d'Infermeria Universitat de Valencia	Yvonne Ford & Volker Gussman-Ford Centre for Communication in Health Care Frankfurt am Main
Associate Partner — Spain	**Associate Partner — Finland**	**Partner — Norway** Bente Børdal
Francisco Javier Barca Duran Escuela Universitaria de Enfermeria Universidad de Extramadura	Irja Saarikorpi Tampereen Terveyden Huolto-Oppilaitos Tampere	Hogskolen i Hedmark Elverum

It is important to note at this stage that events outside of the control of the project team were to play an important part in determining the future of the work. In March 1996 Humberside County Council was abolished as part of the re-organization of local government instituted by Westminster. For a while the prospects for this, and other European projects, looked to be uncertain. It was clear that the European Awareness initiative was unlikely to be adopted by the smaller successor authorities and approaches were made to the University of Hull. This resulted in a transfer of the project together with existing personnel as part of the Curriculum Development Unit. The transfer of project 'ownership' in the eyes of the European Commission, the prospect of redundancy (happily averted) for some of the personnel involved and no less than three physical locations for the Curriculum Development Unit have tested the management strategies to the full. The forbearance of the partners during these difficult months was an essential ingredient for any success that might be achieved.

An outline of project planning methodology

The project planning methodology largely devolved from the management and evaluation structures required on the application form. To some extent the structure of the form rather led the project at this stage, rather than the other way round. It seemed essential to propose and staff (in theory) a number of groups which might conceivably interact and make the project a reality. These groups currently manage the project and their meetings and day to day interactions are essential components of whatever has so far been achieved and essential pre-requisites for the success of the remainder of the project:

The Steering Group

This group guides the general direction and purpose of the project and also provides some expertise and consultancy. It comprises:

Project Co-ordinators (Ray Kirtley and Carol Ludvigsen)
Language Consultant (Josephine Holden)
Project Worker (Kim Dent-Brown)
Technical Co-ordinator (Ian Dolphin)
An adviser on the Training of Nurses (provides knowledge of requests from the user group at Community level). This position is occupied by Joan Kemp from the University of Hull
A representative from the Humberside Training and Enterprise Council (provides expertise on training needs and business applications). This position is occupied by Martin Pinnick.

The group meets at about four monthly intervals during the course of the project. Each meeting has an agenda and is minuted. The group has the function of directing the work of the project at a local level and ensuring that the project targets are met. The group is joined by others from time to time – for example by Michael Lenahan from the UK Leonardo office.

The Management Group

This consists of:
The **Technical and Linguistic Co-ordinator**s who:

- agree system requirements for gathering resources
- are responsible for software quality control

- organize the processing of resource material into digital format
- are responsible for feedback from field trials and subsequent modification

and

The **Project Co-ordinators** (2) who:

- are responsible for the logistic planning of the project
- organise trials, meetings and dissemination
- liaise with all outside agencies
- are responsible for the financial management of the project
- assume the role of the Project Worker for the UK but in addition will oversee the clinical integrity of the project

A further and vital group were the **Project Partners and Associate Partners** without whom the project could not have proceeded.

An outline of project implementation and monitoring

The project divided itself into a number of stages. These were predetermined by the eventual product (an interactive CD-ROM and language learning materials). However, the problem with implementation, from the point of view of the co-ordinators, was that so much of the implementation was devolved. This was inevitable given the multi-faceted nature of the project but the number of players, each with their own specialisms, made it a difficult workplan to direct and to keep to schedule. The activities for the first year of the project gives some clues to this complexity:

1. Revision of workplan and budget

The workplan and timetable were revised early in 1996 in consequence of a reduction in funding and also because of the shorter timescale. In doing this the management group and partners respected the requirements of the contract but had to introduce some modifications notably to the number of scenarios on the CD-ROM.

The original aim of the project was to produce 10 short interactive scenarios on CD-ROM which would be useful to healthcare professionals who needed to acquire vocational language skills. At a meeting with the partners in early March 1996 it became clear that differences in the health services of the countries concerned made it impossible to find 10 replicable situations for four countries. However, it was comparatively easy to extend the functions and usefulness of a smaller number of scenarios through a more complex set of material on screen. The combination of this practical restraint coupled with the reduced budget led to the following scenarios being agreed for development countries. These were then scripted:

Scenario 1
Admitting an elderly patient for a medical purpose into a hospital.

Scenario 2
A home assessment of an adult stroke patient after discharge.

Scenario 3
Introducing a new student into a ward environment (setting the scene, who is in charge, where is the clinic).

Scenario 4
Handover situation between two nurses discussing a mentally ill patient.

Scenario 5
Health promotion in school. The role of the nurse looking at the issue of smoking using questions and answers.

2.   Meetings of project partners

There have been two meetings of the whole project group. The first took place in March 1996 in Hull, the second in March 1997, again in Hull. In each instance we were fortunate to be joined by one of the Associate Partners. The purpose of the meetings was to:

- Collect background information from each partner;
- Assess the current state of technology for each partner;
- Outline the roles of partners and co-ordinator;
- Decide upon the target group(s) for the finished product within our health services;

- Make decisions on the number and complexity of scenarios;
- Make decisions on the location, personnel and scripting of scenarios
- Agree a timetable of activities: locations, shooting, deployment of personnel;
- Make clear the allocation of funding (including own funding) and the allowable costs;
- Review work on a demo CD-ROM;
- Agree transcription and translation details;
- Draw up a formal agreement;
- Draw up an agreement about commercialisation of the product.

3. Filming of scenarios

Filming scenarios – Spain
This took place in June 1996. The location was in and around the hospital in Valencia where our partner Ramon Camano-Puig works in nurse education. The film crew was accompanied by Carol Ludvigsen from the Health Trust.

Filming scenarios – UK
This took place in July 1996. The locations were a number of Health Service centres in the Hull area. The film crew was accompanied by Kim Dent-Brown from the Health Service.

Filming scenarios – Germany and Norway
This took place in a single session in August 1996. The locations were in and around Frankfurt am Main where our partner Yvonne Ford operates as a language trainer for health specialists and around the town of Elverum in Norway where Bente Børdal works in nurse education.

4. Initial editing sessions

Following the fiming sessions it became clear that the editing of the material, both for the CD and the accompanying video, would present Curriculum Development with some difficulties in choosing the most appropriate material in linguistic and vocational terms. Each partner was approached and arrangements were made for them to come to Hull on an individual basis to work with Kim Dent-Brown and the programmers. This took place between November 1996 and January

1997. By the end of these sessions we had created the necessary material for both the CD and video:

- 1.5 minutes of video ready for capture, per scenario in each language;
- 7 minutes of soundtrack for the CD, per scenario in each language;
- Up to 20 minutes of video per partner.

5. Work on the CD ROM

The preparation of interactive framework has taken place at Curriculum Development (part of the University of Hull). A framework has been prepared to accept the video clips, interactive sessions, translations and exercises devised by the project group and now captured on video and tape.

6. Work of the language consultant

The language consultant joined the project in September 1996. Josephine Holden has a background in language teaching but is currently doing research work on the use of interactive materials for the independent learner. She has worked with each partner on the priorities for vocational language learning for nurses from elsewhere in the EU. She has also worked on the activities which appear on disk and which will be supported by paper materials and glossary.

7. Collection of cultural material

At the meeting in March 1996 it was agreed that a common framework should be drafted for the cultural/workplace information section. The Spanish partner agreed to take on this task. It is to this framework that we intend to attach cultural items.

The conclusions and outcomes of the project

This has been, and continues to be, a complex project compared with some of the others which have been co-ordinated by Curriculum Development. It brings our linguistic and software specialists in contact with the unfamiliar world of the health sector. At this stage in the project it seems clear that a product will be produced and possibly commercialised. There are however a number of question marks still hanging over the final outcomes:

Will the product have a ready market in the healthcare sector? Our initial market analyses have been too superficial to give a conclusive answer to this question.

Will the concept attract further funding from the European Commission? We have plans to extend the number of languages involved and even to widen the sectoral appeal however the pressure to complete existing projects on time is a constant deterrent to getting involved in more!

Will the project make any impact on the linguistic barriers that prevent nurses moving confidently within the EU in search of work?

Will the project have real impact on the healthcare sector?

We may have a superficial answer to these final questions once DiNET is completed but it will require a further project to quantify and assess the real impact of the work.

Dissemination

Dissemination is a priority for most European Commission funded projects and it is prudent to set aside time and resources to make this a definitive part of the project. The Commission requires a clear strategy in this area and will expect to see dissemination products and outcomes from the very outset of the project.

In the DiNET project dissemination activities have become more demonstrable in the middle section of the workplan as the opportunity arose to use the demonstration CD-ROM and materials. The list of activities below does show a dissemination presence almost from the start of the project but it must be admitted that early activities were relatively 'low key'. The partners were encouraged to participate in this process and this was one of the aims of having the leaflet available in all of the project languages.

The dissemination activities too were useful, not only to explain the achievements of the project but also to mention some of the pedagogical and operational problems posed by the project. Chief among these was the understanding that the starting point of language learners varies enormously. Intuition and experience told us that the starting point of an English learner of Norwegian is vastly different to a Norwegian learner of English. It was therefore difficult to establish a base level for language teaching. A further lesson is that four-way language learning is a huge undertaking and available funding limits the range of language that can be presented. Most similar packages are two-way. This created a huge translation task and also had major implications for determining the language of instruction.

1. Project leaflet

A project leaflet was produced by Curriculum Development. At the same time a list of recipients was proposed and was compiled by the partners for their own healthcare systems and by the co-ordinator for wider circulation. Recipients included all nurse training establishments in the countries concerned and all policy makers and professional bodies for this sector. The leaflet was later available in Finnish (thanks to the assistance of one of the associate partners) and in French.

2. Articles in professional journals and references to the project in other publications

The project has been mentioned in recent articles:

The Health Service Journal: 'Foreign Exchange' by Carol Ludvigsen (January 1997).
Eurohealth: 'How healthcare organizations can respond to and benefit from the European agenda' by Carol Ludvigsen (Vol 3. No. 1, Spring 1997)
Nurse Education Today: 'Enhancing nurse mobility in Europe: a case for language skills' by Carol Ludvigsen (April 1997).

3. Attendance at conferences, seminars and workshops

The project featured in two local conferences on European issues and the Health Service. This was in terms of a presentation by one of the project team:

Hull and Holderness Community Health Trust, March 1996.
East Riding Health Trust, December 1996.
    The project is also due to feature at conferences which are connected with language learning and the use of technology rather than

the health service. These are the EUROCALL conference in Dublin (September 1997) and the CALL conference in Exeter in the same month.

The Spanish partner also demonstrated the CD-ROM at Health Service conferences in both Valencia and Barcelona in April 1997.

4. Websites

The project has a web page on the Curriculum Development site with hypertext links to explanations of the project in the languages of the partnership.

http://www.hull.ac.uk/Hull/CTLS_web/currdev/top.htm

Jargonbuster

Note: we have tried as far as possible to avoid using jargon or complicated terminology in this book. However, it is impossible to find your way through the world of project management without an explanation of some of the terms commonly used, even though they may refer to techniques you do not select for use in your projects. The list below is not exhaustive, but provides an introduction.

Baseline Plan
The final plan for the project, agreed with the funding agency or sponsor before implementation can begin.

Benchmarking
See Appendix 3 of Section 1. Benchmarking consists of scrutinizing and comparing the way things are done in one (usually model) organization with the practice in your own.

Brainstorming
A simple technique for generating ideas and encouraging creative thinking with a group. See the Toolkit for instructions on how to do it.

Cause and Effect Diagram
This is also known as a Fishbone Diagram because of its appearance. An example is provided in the Toolkit section.

Critical Path
The sequence of events and activities essential to your project. Plotting

these is usually done by Critical Path Analysis (CPA) or Critical Path Method (CPM), techniques which use graphical representations of a project to schedule activities.

Deming

W. Edwards Deming was probably the most famous exponent of the philosophy known as Total Quality Management. Born in the USA in 1900, he was originally a mathematician and statistician who became involved in the post-war Japanese 'economic miracle' and was subsequently credited with originating many of the ideas underpinning it. His approach was to focus on systematic and continuous improvement of the product. His ideas were developed within manufacturing industries but have since been modified and widely applied within the service sector. See Appendix 2 in Section 1 for information about TQM.

Fishbone Diagram

See Cause and Effect Diagram.

Forcefield Analysis

A technique used to focus thought processes on the factors which can affect an activity or project positively or negatively – driving forces or restraining forces. The power or strength of these factors is assessed and ranked accordingly, and is usually represented as a graph.

GANTT Chart

Named after Henry Gantt, an industrial engineer who invented the technique. It is a horizontal chart with the steps or stages ('milestones') of a project represented as lines on the chart, seen against the timescales available.

SWOT Analysis

SWOT stands for Strengths, Weaknesses, Opportunities and Threats. It is a technique used for viewing projects or other activities and preparing for eventualities, and usually undertaken as a group exercise.

Select bibliography

Project Management

Project Management. Harvey Maylor, published by Pitman Publishing 1996.
Project Leadership. Wendy Briner, Michael Geddes and Colin Hastings. Gower Publishing Company, 1994.
Planning Projects. Trevor L. Young. The Industrial Society, 1993.
Leading Projects. Trevor L. Young. The Industrial Society, 1993.
Implementing Projects. Trevor L. Young. The Industrial Society, 1993.

Total Quality Management and related issues

The Deming Management Method: the Complete Guide to Quality Management. Mary Walton, published by Mercury, 1992.
Total Quality Management: the Key to Business Improvement. A Peratec executive briefing. Published by Chapman and Hall, 1994.
The Quality Gurus: what can they do for your company? One of the DTI's Managing in the '90s series of booklets. Published by the Department of Trade and Industry, 1991
BS 5750/ISO 9000/EN 29000: 1987: a positive contribution to better business. An executive guide to the use of national, international and European quality standards. A DTI booklet, published by the Department of Trade and Industry, 1993.

General

Developing Management Skills for Europe. David Whetton, Kim Cameron and Mike Woods. Published by Harper Collins, 1994.

Index